MEDITATE THE POUNDS AWAY

How I Met My Weight Loss and Wellness
Goals Through Meditation

by:

Suki S. Miller

Copyright © 2015 Suki S. Miller
All rights reserved.

ISBN-10: 0692500960
ISBN-13: 978-0692500965

This book is dedicated to all of those who have struggled with weight loss, doing the right things, without the results. It's time to make it happen!
.

CONTENTS

	Acknowledgments	i
	Preface	1
	Introduction	7
PART 1	The Medical Journey	11
Chapter 1	My Story	12
Chapter 2	A Strong Foundation for Wellness	19
Chapter 3	Proactive Wellness	23
PART II	The Mental and Spiritual Journey	30
Chapter 4	What is Meditation?	31
Chapter 5	Components of a Successful Meditation	35
Chapter 6	Your Home is your Wellness Spa	47
Chapter 7	Meeting your Guides	51
Chapter 8	Believing	59
Chapter 9	Visualization, Imagery and Affirmations	63
Chapter 10	Meditations	69
Chapter 11	Putting It All Together	86
Appendix I	Cholesterol	89
Appendix II	Hormones	91

Appendix III	Injectable & Liposomal Supplements	94
Appendix IV	Quick Start to Meditation	101
Appendix V	Gratitude Exercises	105
Appendix VI	Reading/Viewing, Products/ Resources	109
	About the Author	114
	Contact Information	115

MY GRATITUDE LIST
(Acknowledgements)

First, I am forever grateful to my husband, best friend and love of my life, Mark, who has been fully supportive of me on my path. We have both continued to benefit from our mutual physical and spiritual journey.

I am grateful to the members of my 'wellness team' who have helped me to learn about spirituality, my body, about my challenges and helped me to brainstorm our way to success.

I'm forever grateful to Mitzi Schardt, MSN, NP who is referred to variously as 'my wellness guru', our integrated medicine provider and with many other accolades. She has tirelessly answered my many questions and has helped me to understand what it is that my body needs and my body wasn't getting, and why. She's become a dear friend.

Gratitude to Dr. Andrew J . Rózsa Ph.D. Licensed psychotherapist with a specialty in Medical Psychology. Dr. Rózsa introduced me to the concept of the mind / body connection and for that, I am eternally grateful. It is the basis of all I have learned in my life since then.

Many thanks to Elissa Bentsen has helped me along my spiritual journey, helping me to address the many challenges I've faced from past life issues, as well as helping me to connect with many of my current guides and many angels and archangels I work with on a daily basis.

As my reiki instructor, Dorothea Delgado was key to helping me connect with my personal guides. It was the first step in my spiritual awakening and she has always been available to help with this. She is an incredibly talented energy worker.

Angie Arkin is another intuitive healer and her path has been an inspiration to me for many years.

While not part of my weight loss journey, Elizabeth Severino has been important to the wellness of our beloved feathered and furry family members. If they are well, then I am well.

Thanks to Michael Haskins for his direction with book formatting, editing and the rest of the nuts 'n' bolts.

I am grateful to my amazing mother, now on the other side, who instilled in me the ability to love myself and others. With my meditation, we speak daily, much like we once did on the telephone.

I am grateful to our dear loving friends, Don and Jeanie Cohen, who have always been supportive of me, of my life and of my endeavors. Jeanie is recently transitioned but I still have her guidance, support and ideas every single day.

I am grateful for and I thank Rose, Joseph, Edward, George and Joel. You're with me all day, every day and it continues to be amazing.

And finally, I send my love and gratitude to you, the readers. I have confidence that you will succeed when all the pieces fall into place.

PREFACE

If someone had told me eight years ago that I would have meditated my way to health, I would have never believed it. But indeed, I've done it!

This is the part where an author tells about her professional qualifications. My qualifications are different than many. I am not a doctor. I am not a chemist. I am not a dietician. I am not an exercise guru, a yogi nor a meditation teacher. I am a manager and I am an artist. My background is in business, marketing / public relations, travel and 'efficiency'. I am just an every-day person with the same struggles that most people have. It took me eight years to get to the point where I am today, but it doesn't need to take that long for you. I want to share my trials and errors and am happy to help you find your direction.

This is the story of my journey from an overweight, unhealthy person to a healthy, normal weight person. There have been many steps in this process, and there was much trial and error. But every step of the process brought me closer and closer to the place where I am today,

So you might ask "Why the lotus" as our cover art? I see it as a symbol of my journey. The lotus has similar meaning in different cultures. Have you ever really paid attention to a lotus flower in all its' brilliance, against the murky water of a pond? This beautiful flower folds it's petals and sinks into the murky pond water every night. The next day, it emerges with the sun, another bright, beautiful reminder that every day is a new day and a new chance to grow and to move forward in life. The flower is so pure and pristine against the pond water and is proof that we are all capable of this type of personal renewal and growth. The ancient Egyptians associated this flower with the sun god and is a symbol of re-awakening and purity. In Buddhism, the lotus is a symbol of rebirth, purity and also spiritual awakening, as well as a desire for enlightenment. In Hinduism, the lotus flower additionally is associated with beauty, fertility, prosperity, spirituality, and eternity .

Since my journey has brought forward in me an awakening and connection with the earth, the ethers and my inner and higher selves, the lotus is the perfect symbol for my process and growth.

I discovered that wellness is not just having a healthy body, nor is wellness a strictly spiritual journey. Our bodies and our spirit are intertwined and interdependent. True wellness requires that the physical body, mental component and spiritual body be in sync. In my case, I tackled the physical issues first and found that while I had made some progress, I wasn't getting close to my goals.

The most miraculous discovery for me was that I control my own body. Once I realized that it took many modalities to walk my path to wellness, my personal physical and spiritual growth moved forward in leaps and bounds.

Meditation is the tool that has given me the total access to the wellness that I'd always strived for, that I never seemed to have before. Granted, success does not happen in a vacuum and you do indeed need to be sure that you have taken advantage of all the diagnostic and informational tools available to you. One cannot simply start to meditate while at the same time, continue bad, unhealthy habits. No, you can't eat fast food, junk food and binge drink and still meditate the weight away. If only it were that simple!

There are untold numbers of books written by dieticians and doctors and proponents of physical exercise. Indeed, you can read many and find that they often offer conflicting views and information. It is confusing to delve through it all and to glean what you feel is important for you. As much as they'd like to think they can do it, no one else can tell you how to live and what the correct path to wellness might be. It is up to you to comb through the information you find and are given, and make decisions that are right for you. What is most important is that you realize that only one person should have control over your wellness and that person is YOU.

Likewise, there are massive numbers of books written on the mental and spiritual components of wellness. These texts explore the many modalities and metaphysical practices and theories that have proven successful to many. And no, I should get this straight right now: This book is NOT about any particular religion and it is NOT about any organized religion or dogma. My purpose is not to convert nor to convince. My path has been to explore many different theories and theologies and my own particular spiritual belief system defies most all known organized religions. My belief system comes from my heart and from my soul, and from my own experiences.

Bottom line? This is your body. This is your life and it is your responsibility and yours alone as to how you want to treat your body, your mind, your heart, to live your life and define your future. The one person who will benefit from your decisions about your body and your wellness will be YOU. Thus it is important to take responsibility right this moment for your body, your health, your life and your future. It is not your doctor's responsibility. It is not the responsibility of your physical trainer. It is not the responsibility of any spiritual leader.

My journey was facilitated by many authors and forward-thinking wellness professionals, as well as the works of individuals who have had exceptional experiences, spiritual awakenings and personal growth.

I am forever indebted to the professional that I call our 'wellness guru', who has helped me to define the path for the physical growth of myself and my husband, as well as for my attitude towards taking personal responsibility for myself. This woman is a medically certified, licensed healthcare practitioner in the field of integrated medicine in South Florida. Because of her, we are now proactive instead of reactive when it comes to our health. I can't stress enough the importance of this in our lives. While she could always write prescriptions like the run-of-the-mill medical doctor out there to address a symptom, her first choice is to instead find the cause of an issue and address it with nutrition and supplementation. She is steadfast in her pursuit of therapies and formulas that might not be generally available. She often works with compounding professionals to design programs that were heretofore unknown. She ignited the spark in me that made me question and research for myself.

My husband and the love of my life, Mark, has always stood by me as I root my way through books and research papers, and as I read into the night sometimes on the subjects of health, wellness and the human body in Western and Eastern medicine, as well as the mind-body connection. While I generally will try my ideas on myself first, he feels he's benefited from all that I've learned. Without his support and steadfast confidence in me, I would have never moved forward to the point where I am today.

Studying non-traditional healing practices and the healing practices of indigenous peoples and other cultures have proven to me that the current state of medical practice in the US is not something that is necessarily compatible with the lifestyles of many of us. In my world, all modalities are explored and valid.

Even with all of the medical and mainstream medical information I'd garnered, I had still hit a wall with my weight loss and wellness goals. And that is when I found that I could make the final jump and meditate those pounds away.

I am thrilled to be able to share my revelations with you and hope that it will spark a journey of discovery for you.

It is my sincere wish that you become a stunning lotus flower, rise from the muddy pond waters and shine in the sun and become your new, healthy, thinner and more spiritual self. here.

INTRODUCTION

Because my path has encompassed two very distinct phases, this book is organized into two sections.

The first details my health and challenges from the past . I have not gone into meticulous detail on medical information because quite honestly, every single person will have varying challenges and differing degrees of illness and health factors. I have given a broad overview of my starting point, the discovery of my own set of health issues, as well as tests and some of the methods we used to correct my problems. Two things are absolutely key in establishing and maintaining wellness in our lives. It comes down to what goes into your body. Healthy food and supplements are a must. But it is important to also address toxins, since an otherwise healthy person can succumb to disease if there are poisons and toxins present.

Diet is the most important component and then thanks to the toxic lifestyles and the toxins in our lives, each person must also discover their own particular challenges with various foods. Nutrition is sorely lacking in today's diet, thanks to chemicals, pesticides and herbicides used in farming and genetically modified foods. The producers of our food want nothing more than to keep the consumer in the dark. They fight every day to keep 'truth in labeling' out of the consumer lexicon. It is up to you to know what you are eating and if the producers of food will not be honest and tell you, then you simply do not have to support these producers and can refuse to buy their products.

Thus, medical testing will give you a good overview of where you are and what your challenges are. I've detailed just a few of the tests that we've used as our guideposts along this journey.

The second section details my mental and spiritual journey, which is far from complete as of this writing.

I found that I eventually had a very clean, healthy diet and health regimen, but without the mental and spiritual component, I was not getting the results I wanted to achieve.

I am detailing some of the more basic tenants of my meditation practice and various foundation beliefs that I work with in my meditation. I am not trying to 'sell' any particular belief system. I don't necessarily adhere to any strict practice or style of meditation. I believe all styles are valid. This is just what has evolved for me to help me with my wellness and weight loss goals.

For those who are already involved in a meditation practice, some of this will be elementary to you and thus, I am attempting to keep this text on point without going too deeply into the basics. You may find that my personal meditation practice varies from yours and of course, I offer my findings so that you can decide if it is helpful for you to adopt some of my methods to your own.

For those who have not devoted time to meditation, I will share some of the basics that for me, have proven most effective. I highly recommend it!

In my world, there is more than just the physical plane in which we live our daily lives. I am aware of my own special spirit guides, many who have been with me my entire life, previous lives and many who come and go as needs arise. I am aware of entities, angels and other beings who have been here for me when I need them - and usually when I don't think that I need them. They're there to help me. They want success for me and they try to keep me from getting in the way of my own success. They want to help us and they love us. But free will dictates that they cannot interfere in our lives. Thus I know that I can call on them at any time. It is important that you find your spirit guides and develop a relationship with them. Learn to listen to them and to their offers of help. Learn to watch for signs that they will send your way. I will share some very brief ideas as to how to meet them and come to know them, if you do not already have knowledge of or a relationship with your guides already.

I will also share some ideas as to how to set the stage for a peaceful space to do your work as you grow spiritually. It is key these days, to develop your sanctuary, a place to renew, refresh and to simply feel safe from the ever-increasing challenges of our society and of our world. If you can refresh nightly, feel safe, nourished and loved in your home, and have a place to build your meditation practice, you will progress with your more physical goals. This space doesn't need to be large. It just needs to be comfortable and peaceful.

The styles of meditation are vast and can be confusing. I will give some more simple steps to begin your meditation practice.

PART 1 THE MEDICAL JOURNEY

Chapter 1

MY STORY

As I am writing this, I am 60 years of age. My weight and health challenges showed up at age 45. I was dating the wonderful man who is now my husband, and we were having the time of our lives! We ate our way though a town with hundreds of eating establishments. It was happy eating and nothing seemed to get in our way. By the time we married in 2003, my weight was the highest it had ever been. It didn't seem to bother him but it did bother me - and it made my previous injuries more difficult to manage. My husband is nothing but positive and supportive.

Prior to that, as a single (divorced) woman, my weight and health were in check, with ethical eating habits, small portions, no red meat, no dairy, lots of veggies and low alcohol consumption.

I mention divorce simply because the first marriage was toxic and offered up an entirely different set of challenges in my life. I married far too young at age 19, and in a matter of months, I was miserable. But young and idealistic, I was determined to make it work anyway. I tried for nineteen years then gave up. He was a verbally and mentally abusive alcoholic, workaholic and compulsive gambler. He called me fat when I was actually fine at age

29, 130 pounds and 5'7". I struggled with my body image because of that. And that was well before women were slammed with Photoshopped magazine covers as an impossible ideal to attain.

In 1992, I suffered a disabling accident and lumbar back injury, resulting in weight gain because my inability to move and a 22% permanent disability rating. After working with a forward-thinking therapist in a work-hardening program that emphasized the mind-body connection, the weight was gone in 12 months - and so was the abusive husband.

I ignored the word 'disability' and continued with my life, doing what I wanted to do while being as active as I could with a badly damaged lumbar area. Being a 'hyper flexible' person, I was prone to sprains all of my life, with a long history of joint sprains (ankle, knee, wrist, elbow). Again, though, with my mind-over-matter thinking, I kept moving forward.

In 2008, I was rear-ended in an accident and that managed to take out the rest of my spine with disk ruptures in the cervical area and even a fracture in the thoracic area. While I tried to keep with my 'move forward' thinking, this actually did bring me to a physical halt. The 'happy weight' had never completely gone away, and with my work being mostly at a desk, any weight loss seemed to stagnate. And now, I had a 33% disability rating.

Simply eating right didn't really seem to do the

trick. Low-calorie eating? My body just held on to the weight as if it were in the starving mode. Low-carb eating? It was good for a month but then nothing further happened.

I was overweight, sluggish, tired, and struggling with the pressure of the weight on my spine, joints and previous injuries. I don't like drugs and refused to take them. The pain was never-ending and eventually it begins to eat at the psyche. I didn't sleep well. I couldn't concentrate and had foggy thinking. I lived in hot-flash world. Oh my! On top of the weight, I was suddenly in menopause hell!

Clearly my health and my life had taken an undesirable detour. Sitting around wasn't the answer. No medical professional had a clue as to where to start. They just want to throw drugs at a symptom and then, they want you to go away. I've found that the majority of western medical practitioners don't want to be reminded that they do not know the answers to big problems. They just know how to treat symptoms. It was time to look for the answers on my own.

While meditation is the key to this book and to my success, I couldn't have gotten very far without a fair assessment of where I began. In my case, working with our integrative health practitioner, my husband and I started with testing. I am blessed to have found a talented, committed practitioner of integrated medicine, Mitzi Schardt. She tested for hormone levels first and then, I began a program known as the Wiley Protocol (detailed in

Appendix II: Hormones), which is natural, compounded bio-identical hormone therapy. This includes a rhythmic cyclic method of hormone delivery, much like your body had done and would do if it could. The hot flashes were gone! The brain fog? Gone! The sleep issues? Gone! And all of the dangers of hormone therapy from the western medical community? For us, we found these were nothing but scare tactics by those who base their opinions on a flawed, obsolete study, and who were not willing to learn anything new or fresh. The laziness of the western medical establishment is alarming.

Our wellness practitioner had also ordered the standard blood panels, lipids and blood chemistry tests. Thyroid levels were checked not for the 'standard' that most medical people go by, but for optimum. The lipid panel she ordered again, was more detailed than the norm and was aimed at treating for optimum health. Obviously she checked weight, blood pressure and other factors.

Not surprisingly, in addition to my weight issue I had elevated blood pressure and some seriously-concerning blood work. What was alarming to me at that time is that I had been eating a very clean, balanced, organic, healthy, GMO-free diet, staying away from red meats, dairy and glutens. I was taking high quality supplements and yet, there were indicators that were of concern to both my Mitzi and myself. The concern was that my nutrition wasn't getting through and my body wasn't processing it.

To find where my nutritional gaps were, we did a

SpectraCell micronutrient assessment, which looks at the nutrients present in your body, how they are functioning and what you are missing. The SpectraCell results indicated a lack of the necessary B-vitamins even though we were taking high-quality B vitamins. So our practitioner ordered various compounded B injectables. My husband and I now do weekly B-12 shots and he does a B-6 as well. I have a negative reaction to the B-6 shots and I take a sublingual Pantethine and an oral folinic acid.

This battery of blood tests showed numerous factors, but the upshot of it was that my body wasn't benefiting from the nutrients, vitamins and minerals that I ingested. This was just the start of our detective work to find out why.

Even though we filter our water to get rid of toxins such as fluoride and metals, even though we filter the air in our home, something was causing my body to reject much of the nutrition that was ingested. And the weight would not go. After several years of annual testing, with constant tweaks in nutrients and supplements, Mitzi was baffled. A few years down the road, one day she said "Mold! It could be mold!" We tested for mold and both my husband and myself were full of mold! This was found to be from hidden black mold Stachybotrys chartarum and Stachybotrys Chlorohalonata which had taken hold in our rented home after Hurricane Wilma flooded it in 2005. The property owner ordered mitigation treatment and the outcome was said to be successful, but it never really left our bodies until two years after we left that property. Now it's totally gone.

Two years ago, I became inexplicably ill, with a

stubborn cough that had taken control of my life. Visits to specialists produced nothing. My blood pressure had gone through the roof. My integrated wellness practitioner felt that after a severe reaction to second hand smoke a year prior, the resulting sinus infection and then the resulting complications from antibiotics that a local physician had prescribed (with massive side effects), my body had never recovered and was reacting. Blood pressure meds were helpful to control the elevated blood pressure, but we weren't getting to the cause. In an attempt to pump up my immune system, I had a glutathione push, and then afterwards, added liposomal vitamin C and liposomal glutathione to our supplementation program. (I share the method and recipe for these amazing supplemental regimes in Appendix III: Injectable and Liposomal Supplements.) Since they don't go through the digestive tract, the liposomals have similar benefits to injectable vitamins. These liposomal supplements are encapsulated so that you end up with over 92% benefit from what you're ingesting, instead of the usual 2% that you can expect from any supplement that goes through your gastrointestinal system. You can purchase these liposomals but they're very expensive and are often made with a soy base, which is a hormone disruptor. Mitzi taught me to make my own, with better ingredients at a very low cost. Since then? Neither I nor my husband have been sick at all.

    A year ago, my weight had only gone down somewhat but there were still far too many stubborn pounds and still some puzzling annual blood work indicators. My dedicated wellness guru, Mitzi, felt that there could be something in the diet to cause my body to react in this way. So I ordered an ALCAT test. This is a blood draw test to ferret out food allergies and sensitivities. Shockingly, I found that I was severely sensitive to many of the healthy foods I ate regularly. Hummus? Who knew? Shrimp and oysters? VERY allergic.

I dropped all of these foods for the recommended six months and re-tested. The blood work, after seven years, was finally coming in line. But still, there was the matter of the weight.

THAT is when I turned to meditation.

Chapter 2

A STRONG FOUNDATION FOR WELLNESS

Any program or goal will only succeed with a strong foundation. Wellness and weight loss are no different. It's important to know where you are before you can move forward. It's the only way to gauge progress.

Nutrition is key to good health. If you don't put good things in, nothing good will come of it. Our food supply has become toxic with the decline of small family farms and the rise of factory farming, GMO foods, pesticides and herbicides. There is also the simple 'bad juju' from the manner in which our food is raised. The truth is, most of the food in this country is not raised ethically. Farm animals do not live a quality life in fresh air and in the sun with natural food. They are raised in cramped, filthy quarters, abused and eating whatever the factory farm feels will fatten them up the fastest. This bad energy translates to our food and then on to those who eat it.

I hope you are aware of the horrors lurking in the food supply in this country. Once the bread basket of the world, US grown grain and crops are now banned in Europe, Asia and other countries across the globe - even Mexico - because of the GMO basis of these crops and other toxins that are part and parcel of the basis for the foods that Americans seem to be willing to eat without even thinking. Advertising continues to tout foods as delicious and nourishing when indeed, these items are 'fake food' with no nutritional value and loaded with toxic ingredients.

Toxins can counteract even the most healthy, nutritious diet. Our lives are filled with toxins at every turn. Most people are totally oblivious to the toxins in their lives, such as chemicals in their furnishings, rugs, fabrics, mattresses and the materials in their home.

Our air and our water are the main source of poisons and toxins that can inhibit wellness and promote disease. Our municipal water sources are full of toxins that can degrade our health with every sip and every shower. Yet our municipalities have been convinced to ADD poisonous manufacturing byproducts to our drinking water by chemical companies. Yes, we all choose to think that our municipal water authority wouldn't poison us, but you have to remember, they are operating based on recommendations that are often obsolete and they have a long-established business relationship with some of the country's most toxic chemical companies. These chemical companies lobby heavily in Washington and that continues to control standards, or lack thereof that are followed nationwide. As an example, fluoride is a poisonous byproduct of aluminum production and was originally sold to municipalities to prevent tooth decay. But there has been no hard evidence that it has done that. There is though, proof that fluoride calcifies the pineal gland in the brain and that it will shut down your thyroid and other necessary glands in your body. These people are not interested in your wellness. It's up to you to do it for yourself and for your family.

Nature can even provide toxins such as airborne molds and poisons that come from the earth.

It goes without saying that the oil and gas industry is one of the biggest polluters of water in this country. Fracking not only ruins water and health, it also ruins property values and families. And how many oil wells are in the waters surrounding the US, and how much marine life is poisoned by these wells and the leaks that can ensue? After the oil spill in the Gulf of Mexico in 2010, surely no one doubts the potential danger to our oceans and our marine food sources any longer.

We breathe toxins every day. The air quality in this country continues to degrade thanks to the presence of lobbyists and corporate money in our legislative branch of government. If it is a choice between profit and bad air, the profit seems to win these days. While the hazards of cigarette smoke and second hand smoke are well documented, there is still not enough done to eliminate this hazard from coming in contact with innocent, healthy people who have no interest in this obsolete, dangerous habit.

I urge you to become a permanent fixture in your legislators' inboxes. If they know that you are watching the way they vote for air and water quality, it could make a difference. We can only hope that our opinions as voters will outweigh the influence of lobbyists and corporate campaign monies.

I will not go into the many dangers in our day-to-day life that can have a profound effect on our wellness, quality of life and longevity. But I do strongly recommend that you do some serious reading on these subjects, or at least, check out the videos online.

Chapter 3

PROACTIVE WELLNESS

Wellness does not just happen in a vacuum. Today we're bombarded with toxins in our air, water and food. Toxins can disable your body's ability to absorb nutrients and to be healthy. There is 'fake food' everywhere, with little or no nutritional value and it is loaded with toxic, unethical ingredients. Ingredients are often hidden. So now we're eating things that are not only unhelpful but can be dangerous. Lives are stressful. A good night's sleep becomes more and more illusive. We get mixed messages from many so-called professionals in many professions. Today XYZ ingredient is bad for you, tomorrow it may be good for you. Society is suffering from an overload of information, good, bad, and confusing.

My mantra is to take responsibility for yourself and your own wellness. This is not an easy task, but it can be done. Information and self-knowledge are the keys to your journey to wellness and weight loss.

I can't begin to stress the importance of proactive wellness as opposed to what most people live and practice, which is reactive. Most people only address their health if they are sick and doctors are more than obliged. Doctors are not trained for wellness and very few have taken the time nor made the effort to learn that wellness is the new paradigm. They have been brain-washed by their professors, the FDA, the drug companies, their associations and the AMA to see health as JUST the treatment of illness and disease. They believe that their way is the only way. On a more insidious note, in the past, doctors have been encouraged to do all they can to squelch other modalities for the "good of their profession." (See the film "Doctored" referenced in Appendix VI.) To their credit, though, today more and more are beginning to embrace options. Sadly, since this is not their training, they are often embracing options that are not necessarily the most up-to-date. Thus, this is another reason that YOU are ultimately responsible for your wellness.

Nature can even provide toxins such as airborne molds and poisons that come from the earth. Please keep all of this in mind as you begin YOUR journey towards proactive wellness.

Proactive Wellness involves two seemingly opposite disciplines: Medical / physical and Mental / metaphysical. These are both important parts of the human experience and work beautifully in sync if managed properly. Both are addressed in this book. Please remember, though, that this is the story of my experience and my journey and I have written it with the intent that others may use learn from my experiences to reach their own weight and wellness goals. I am in no way trying to tell you how to live your life. My hope is that my struggles and my discoveries will help you to move forward with your personal growth.

I am obliged of course, to add this legal disclaimer: This content is not intended to be a substitute for professional medical advice, diagnosis, or treatment. If you think you may have a medical emergency, call your doctor, go to the emergency department, or call 911 immediately

Now, onward!

Step One: What do YOU see as your limitations both mental and physical? Make a list of what you see as your problems, symptoms, and challenges. This list might include "Inability to get a good night's sleep" or "Overweight" or "Tired" or "Distracted". The list can be long but it should be complete. Once you have your list, then it's time to find the right team to help you with these challenges.

Step Two: Start to research your problems. You might find that a drink or two before bedtime is sabotaging your sleep. You might find that your cravings for snacks, sweets, drinks and other unhealthy food is undermining your weight goals. You could find that your hormones are running amok. Your thyroid could be under-performing and may require further investigation. GOOGLE is your friend! (More about that later.) In your favorite browser using your favorite search engine, specifically type in what you wish to learn about. Then read, read, read!

Step Three: You will more than likely find a number of books and websites that include information on your concerns. Read them and then, it's time for you to decide if the information presented feels right for you. It's always important to reflect on the source of the information you read. Many articles are written with an eye to promoting specific products, individuals or organizations. While this doesn't mean the information you read is invalid, it does mean that you should assign appropriate weight to the information.

Step Four: Find an integrated medicine practice or practitioner that will meet your needs. This may not be a simple process. You may have to visit a few to find someone who feels right to you. You may have to travel some distance to find the right practitioner, as we did. However, we found that the travel and time invested in our search was well worth it when we finally saw results. You should look for someone who thinks outside the box. Your usual internist or general practitioner is going to be focused on symptoms and on 'treatment' rather than 'prevention. This is not the person you need right now. These medical people are useful when you have an emergency but when you are totally focused on wellness, they are not going to understand. They'll sit with you a short time, then rush you away to the billing window with a script in hand if possible.

The first thing I ask a practitioner is if they're able to work in partnership with me as a client/patient. I've found that many are deep in a God-complex where they expect total compliance. This is not the type of person you need in this journey. Ask the practitioner about their philosophy towards wellness. Ask what specific modalities they feel most comfortable with. Ask about specific modalities that you have an interest in after you've done your own research and reading. Watch their reactions. And at the risk of putting a negative spin on this part of your search, just be alert for a condescending attitude or an attitude of dismissal. "This is not the droid that you are seeking!"

It is important to know when a practitioner is not the right team member for your growth and wellness team. Their personal appearance and their philosophies will become evident very quickly when you talk to them. A doctor who sells weight loss products such as shakes and pre-packaged meal plans in his/her office is not someone who understands balance and nutrition. A doctor who is herself/himself obese is someone who is not able to ascertain the answers for themselves, much less for others. A doctor who is known to prescribe diet pills? Not your guy! A doctor who herself goes under the knife for stomach reduction surgery is someone whose philosophy is not right for you.

My husband and I have encountered doctors who seem to resent a well-informed, engaged patient. In asking questions or expressing opinions, we've had several doctors make a snide, condescending comment such as "And where did you hear that? Google?" Seriously? One that is threatened by Google or any other search engine is no different that someone who feels threatened by libraries. With one doctor, we persisted in describing a severe side effect to a drug he had prescribed after my husband's surgery to repair accident damage to his clavicle. The doctor had indicated that it was not a known side effect. Interestingly enough, in his attempt to disprove us, HE Googled it on his cell phone in the office and immediately, found that we were indeed correct and he was wrong. I like to think that we have occasionally educated a doctor or two over the years.

A doctor recommend breast reduction surgery to me when I had inflamed cartilage in my rib area from learning to play golf. I felt this was outrageous and of course, did not take his advice. Once I knew that it was a cartilage / connective tissue problem, I found that rest along with hot and cold compresses took care of the problem within a short time and now, of course, without the extra weight, I couldn't imagine having that problem again.

The cut 'n' drug approach to medicine is NOT what you need if you wish to lose weight in a healthy manner and keep it off. I truly believe that you will appreciate your journey and your accomplishments if do not take short cuts. Surgery is a tragic and dangerous shortcut and you will not learn the right way to take care of yourself in this manner.

Then I met the integrated medical professional that we work with now, Mitzi Schardt. Her approach was to do blood testing to see what was happening in my body, what my body lacked, and what my body may have too much of, besides the obvious fat. She made it very clear that her first requirement of a client / partner was for me to take responsibility for my own health. Interestingly, our local internist scoffed at that approach!

Step Five: Once you've found your practitioner / wellness partner and perhaps other team members, the detective work begins. It is often a process of elimination, but diligence on your part and on the part of your wellness partner will indeed pay off.

Step Six: When all your testing indicates that the obvious nutritional and hormonal problems have been solved, then it's time to move forward.

Step Seven: Now it's time to put your mind, your spirit, your heart and your soul to work! Now THAT is what I call a team!

PART 2

THE MENTAL AND SPIRITUAL JOURNEY

Chapter 4

WHAT IS MEDITATION?

Meditation is an ancient practice that goes back to the earliest of times and it is a means to quiet your mind, listen to your spirit, to your heart and to your angels and guides. You connect to the earth, to the heavens, to your core, to your spirit and using any number of techniques, you will learn lessons from your spirit and your guides about energy, love, patience, generosity and forgiveness. Once you have become comfortable with the meditation technique you choose, then you can fine tune it and begin to set intentions for your meditation sessions.

Meditation has been used for healing for centuries. However, one of the most fascinating accounts of use of meditation for healing is quite recent. In 2003, at the age of 37, Tibetan Lama Phakyab Rinpoche had immigrated to the United States. He suffered from diabetes, as well as a form of tuberculosis and because of the diabetes and associated diseases, had developed gangrene in his right foot and leg. Various doctors in New York recommended amputation. The Rinpoche consulted with the Dali Lama, his teacher, who suggested that he use his skills at Tsa Lung meditation to heal himself, and then teach others the value of this ancient art. For a year, the Rinpoche meditated. He would devote every day to meditation, breaking only for meals, taking no medication and getting a good nights' sleep. After nine months, the liquid from his leg began to clear and the ever-present swelling went down. A month later, he could walk with crutches and before the end of a year, he could walk unassisted. And his diabetes and other diseases had disappeared. A group of doctors at New York University have been studying the Rinpoche's brain, to get a better idea of how this medication had such a curative effect. This is an example of meditation's curative effect in an extreme state. Imagine what it can do for our everyday ailments!

If you are experienced in meditation, then you only need to begin to add specific visualizations, intentions and suggestions to your meditation to begin to take control of your body, your weight and your health, and to ask for specific assistance from guides and angels who are specialists in the matters where you need help.

If you are not experienced in meditation, you can research the many styles of meditation. While there are many ways of getting to the proper state for effective meditation, I am going to share my particular method, complete with visualizations, aids, specific guides and angels and spirits.

The most important thing to remember about meditation is that it is a practice and it should be done daily, without fail. To me, meditation is now as important to me as washing my face or brushing my teeth. Many people find that they meditate better at night but for me, it has become an integral part of my morning. The word 'practice' is defined as "to perform an activity or exercise repeatedly or regularly in order to improve or maintain proficiency." However, it is important not to attach concrete expectations to your practice. I often have days where I do not feel my meditation has been effective and that means that I have attached my own expectations. Yes, I'm still working on that part.

Meditations can last from 10 minutes to hours. Mine have progressed from 20 minutes, to 30 minutes, to an hour and now on weekends when I have the luxury of time, perhaps an hour and a half. I have friends who have two hour meditation sessions every morning. If my day is particularly stressful, I try to do a mini-meditation mid-afternoon that will last about 20 minutes.

As I've developed my own personal meditation style, I have begun to use it for my health, healing, wellness, my weight, my abundance, my relationships with family members both here on this plane and on the other side, my pets and my personal lifetime goals.

To find what feels right to you, I recommend that you read Wikipedia's definition of meditation, and then read any number of 'beginner meditation' how-to's online. I particularly like Gaiam Life's "Meditation 101 techniques". Per this article, short term benefits of meditation include lower blood pressure and heart rate, less anxiety, less stress, deeper relaxation. I have noticed that I am no longer as angry in traffic and in political discussions. And yes, my blood pressure is now perfect. (The question on that point is whether it has to do with the weight loss or the meditation. In my case, since the weight loss has finally come because of the meditation, I credit both.)

You might also consider working with a gifted intuitive healer, teacher, energy worker or psychic a few times to help you to find the most comfortable method of meditation for you. They can often help you with the relaxation process and some basic visualizations. Of course, be sure to phone or email ahead and ask if they can help you with this. Some prefer to jump right into healing without the teaching component. You will find a few that I recommend in the section Appendix VI: Reading, Viewing, Products and other Life Resources.

You may choose to meditate sitting or lying down. I often choose to use crystals in my meditation as a point of focus and to help align my chakras. From time to time, I use aromatherapy sprays and mists as well.

You will design your own program, but I am sharing my experiences with you simply as a starting point..

Chapter 5

COMPONENTS OF A SUCCESSFUL MEDITATION

Before you jump into meditation, it is important to set the stage for success. Obviously, a wellness-directed lifestyle is a must. And while one can theoretically meditate anywhere, I have never found that to be the case for me.

A peaceful home or other stress-free location is a must:

Home is not just a place to eat and sleep. Your home can be your own personal spa. I'll devote a chapter to turning your home into an inviting, restful escape. This isn't something that occurs organically. You usually have to work at creating a peaceful space for your life. Pets are an excellent way to manage stress in your life and their unconditional love sets the tone for your daily life. While many pets love meditation, rambunctious younger cats and dogs will be distracting. While there is endless kvetching outside the door to my room, I give myself at least an hour without my little darlings every morning when it's time to meditate.

Make yourself comfortable:

Many mediate sitting on a sofa or chair, with feet on the ground and arms at their side, or hands on their legs, with palms up. Because of my back issue, and for my use of crystals, I prefer to meditate lying down. I use a comfortable pillow under my head and because of my back (and the amount of time I'm lying in the same position), I put one or two pillows under my knees. Make sure the temperature is comfortable. A light cover is good if the room is warm, or if it's cooler, then perhaps a bit more in the way of covering is good. You can meditate with clothing or without.

Aromatherapy:

I personally use a small collection of aromatherapy sprays to once again, help to set my intention for my meditation. Two resources are noted in the Appendix VI: Reading, Viewing, Products and other Life Resources. I use a couple of sprays from time to time that are attuned to various archangels, spirits and guides. My go-to sprays are for Archangel Michael, Archangel Raphael, Archangel Ariel, and Lakshmi. Other complimentary sprays are Smudge In Spray, Miracles and Guardian Angel sprays. I lightly spray the area where I will meditate and lightly mist myself from above, concentrating the entire time on the intention that will be evoked with that particular spray. I also use these sprays at night before bedtime, to invoke my angels and healers to promote rest.

Your Chakras:

Chakras are the eight main energy centers of our etheric body and the chakra system plays an important role in many of the practices of religions throughout the world. Each center is associated with specific organ(s) and with the energies necessary to run the organ(s) and to keep the energy flowing along the spine. Each chakra has a color associated with it. It is very important to keep this energy flowing and balanced within your body and in your metaphysical field. Amazon has a number of excellent books available on the chakra system.

Again, I won't be going into the details and specifics of each chakra and will give a small overview of each. I highly recommend doing your personal research on the subject of the chakras, since personal research will help you to define the chakras in a manner that is most meaningful to you.

The first chakra is the Base or Root Chakra. The color associated with this chakra is red and it is an intense, spinning energy in the lower region of your body at the base of your spine. This chakra is related to Earth and thus, the basics of survival and life. Your instincts of self preservation, survival and trust are rooted in this area. This is the chakra that grounds you to the earth, keeps basic bodily functions going and helps you to remain in the physical world. The organs that are connected to the base or root chakra are prostate, kidneys, bladder and spine.

The second chakra is the Sacral Chakra, located slightly below the navel. The color associated with this chakra is orange and this is related to your sexuality, relationships, ability to feel empathy, pleasure, emotions, and to feel connection to yourself and to others. This is the center of your inward feeling of self, of your ability to make and maintain relationships, and your ability to detect and feel emotions of others. The organs that are connected to the sacral chakra are your reproductive organs.

The third chakra is the Solar Plexus, located slightly above the navel. The color associated with this chakra is yellow and it is all about power, joy and energy. This chakra is the center of motivation, self-identification, the power over your relationship with others. The Solar Plexus gives you the desire to express individuality, allows you to master your own light, follow your own path, and to stand steady and strong on your own. Strengthen your Solar Plexus to learn to process unrefined emotions and personal power. This center gives us the sense of complete satisfaction and contentment. The organs that are ruled by the Solar Plexus are the pancreas, stomach, liver, and gall-bladder.

The fourth chakra is the Heart Chakra, located in the center of the chest. The colors associated with this chakra are green or pink. This chakra is exactly what you think it should be: Love, devotion, compassion, balanced emotions, an open heart and love for self and others. The Heart Chakra allows one to experience unconditional love and affection and spiritual growth. This is the bridge or connecting point between the lower and higher energies in the chakra system, and is where our true spirit and true self reside. The organs ruled by the heart chakra are the heart, liver, lungs, and the circulatory system.

The fifth chakra is the Throat Chakra, located at the base of the throat. The color is a bright or rich blue. Not surprisingly, this is the center for communication, intuition, creativity, sound and self expression. You speak your truth and hear the truth through this energy center. This is the center that controls your thyroid gland, as well as your throat, upper lungs, arms and digestive track. Thus, for the purposes of this book and your weight-loss meditation, it is important to work with this chakra as much as possible.

The sixth chakra is known as the Third Eye and is located in your forehead. The color associated with this chakra is indigo. My persistent meditation practice has activated my Third Eye and it is a physical sensation, as well as the sensation of intuition and perception. In working with and developing your third eye chakra, you will find that you have more power over yourself, your future, your decisions and your imagination. This center controls your pituitary gland, spine, lower brain, nose, ears and left eye. Again, this is a particularly important chakra when it comes to weight loss and wellness, since it works with the pituitary gland (which works with the thyroid gland) and of course, your brain. Your brain is highly important in this process because what you believe WILL happen. When the third eye opens, you are experiencing spiritual awakening. If your brain embraces your goals, your body will follow. What you visualize using your third eye, will come to pass. The third eye also is the seat of compassion and forgiveness. The path to weight loss and controlling your body involves a great deal of compassion for yourself and forgiveness for your past decisions. One of the roadblocks to the opening of the third eye is our modern lifestyle. At the center of this chakra is said to be the pineal gland in your brain. Mankind in the so-called 'civilized world' has lost much of it's connection to intuition and the very real gifts of clairvoyance, clairsentience and clairaudience because the pineal gland has become calcified by the fluoride in our water and foods. Get rid of the fluoride to activate your pineal gland!

The seventh chakra is the Crown Chakra and is located at the top of the head. The color associated with this chakra is violet. This is the center of intelligence, divine wisdom, bliss and connection with spirit. The crown chakra represents the highest level of consciousness and enlightenment. Here, all chakras are brought together to manifest the properties and qualities of each. We all hope to achieve the goal of mastering the lower vibrational aspects of our being, reside in and rejoice in the full awareness that we are spiritual beings so that we can living the ultimate human experience. This chakra works with the pineal gland, upper brain and right eye, thus this too will have a beneficial influence on your weight loss goals.

An eighth chakra is not generally addressed, but indeed, this chakra does exist and is known as the Star Chakra or Seat of the Soul. The color for this chakra is a brilliant white light. It is located above the top of the head, above the crown chakra and is situated above the highest point of the physical body. Imagine it to be about six inches

Crystals:
       I use crystals to help direct my focus to my chakra areas. If you are drawn to crystals, for starters, you can easily pick up an inexpensive collection of chakra crystals to place on your chakras during meditation. Tumbled stones often will work as well as raw stones.

       Prior to the start of my meditation, I lay crystals in the corresponding chakra areas on my body. There are many, many choices to use in this process, so I recommend getting to know your crystals. When shopping for crystals, hold a crystal and see how it feels to you. My choices for crystals come from many years of collecting and 'knowing' crystals. Even as a small child, I was never happier than digging in the earth, looking for rocks and stones that excited my imagination.

My choices:

       Base Chakra - I place this actually under my body at the base of my spine. I use a lovely, flat, heavy hematite stone since it is particularly grounding.

       Sacral Chakra - I place this slightly below my naval and use a carnelian. If I'm having a monthly issue with cramps, I also add some bloodstones on either side of the carnelian.

       Solar Plexus - For whatever reason, I feel the need

to 'load this area up' with crystals. I use mainly citrine and often use several. I also add a Herkimer Diamond to amplify this energy.

Heart Chakra - I use a rose quartz carved in the shape of an arrowhead. I also add a Herkimer Diamond if for any reason I feel the need to amplify this energy.

Throat Chakra - Now this is a bit of a balancing act. I start with a kyanite blade, and then use on either side, a pair of sodalite crystals. I often add a Herkimer here also. Ok, so I'm a bit of an over-achiever.

On the third eye, I use either an amethyst or a diamond. I simply use my engagement ring in this area since to me, the diamond represents more than the stone itself. Again, the over-achiever in me feels more is better, so I often put a tumbled amethyst on either side of my head.

At the crown chakra, I have a nice, triangular piece of sugalite that I use.

Finally, at the star chakra, I often add a clear, large Herkimer Diamond about two to four inches above my head, to represent communication with the star chakra.

Again, you may choose your own stones and crystals if you choose to work with them. It is very important to keep your crystals clean with clear energy, I use Smudge In Spray from TheCrystalGarden.com. It's far easier and safer for your crystals than other methods.

You may notice I used Herkimer Diamonds often. These serve to amplify the energy of other stones and also can substitute for any stone that you wish it to stand for. This is not an actual diamond, but a very clear, double-terminated quartz that originates from upstate New York.

If I have any particular aches or pains that may distract me during my meditation, I have several crystals that I place in the area to soothe the problem. If I'm having a back problem in the area of kidneys, I have two very smooth, flat honey calcite 'palm stones' that I slide under the area that is aching. A crystal that is helpful for me for the pain in my hip flexor is a large piece of fluorite. And a great all-purpose crystal for all aches and pains is again, the Herkimer diamond.

A crystal that I have found to be particularly helpful when reaching a meditative state is Moldavite. You can use on your heart chakra, your third eye or your crown chakra. Moldavite, by the way, seems to be a favorite of Archangel Raphael.

Sounds:

Because I am easily distracted by noises, like many people, I choose music for my meditation. I use music downloaded to my iPhone and ear buds. Music is also a good way to manage my meditation time without actually opening my eyes and looking at my watch. My chosen track is a 30 minute track and I set to repeat, so I can be aware of the time frame. Choose something that resonates with you. There are multitudes of CD's and music files for meditation. iTunes is an excellent resource and it allows you to listen to about 90 or 120 seconds so you can decide if the music is right for you. There is a vast array and it's important to find something that not only relaxes you, but triggers your mind's ability to go within. Many like orchestral pieces, electronic music, chimes, ringing of glass bowls and other tones. Sometimes the music isn't really music. I have found for me, that the NASA Voyager Space Sounds / Jupiter is a excellent basic. I've used it continuously and now, when the track starts, it is far easier to get into my meditation mode. Should you be drawn to space sounds, you should listen to the bytes on iTunes through headphones or ear buds to discover your reaction. I have a friend who is very drawn to the sounds of Neptune. The sounds of nature are also conducive to meditation. Wild birds, mountain streams, the sound of waves on a beach or a mountain rain storm work well for some.

Guides and Angels:

Now, the most important parts of my meditation are my guides and angels. I ask them to join me and I ask for their assistance and guidance. The universe is full of guides, angels, archangels and ascended masters. For me, the best resource has been Doreen Virtue's "Archangels and Ascended Masters". I highly recommend this book. It will help you to find the angels and guides that can be of service to you. They honestly want to serve you but because everything is based on free will, you must ask for their help.

We each have our own personal guides. When

you begin to meditate, you can ask your guides to identify themselves and ask their names. Perhaps you can see them. I'm more clairsentient than clairvoyant and I end up seeing mainly colors, but I learned the names of my guides many, many years ago, shortly after my Reiki Masters certification. It was just a sudden 'knowing'. If this information is not coming to you readily, you might consider working with an intuitive healer or energy worker to help you discover your personal guides. They're definitely there. But it helps to develop a personal relationship if you can visualize them or hear them or know their names and purpose. I have found them to be with me all the time, and they do the work for many of the archangels and ascended masters.

As you develop your meditation style, you will become comfortable with your guides. You will know when they're there, and you can ask their help at any time whatsoever.

Intention:

It is important to set your intention for your meditation sessions. Your general intention may be that you intend for your body to be healed, or that you intend to reach an optimum weight of x pounds.

Craft your intention as if it has already happened. "Thank you for helping me to solve my XYZ problem" or "thank you for healing my injury". Put some emotion into it. Feel the joy at achieving your cure or experiencing the healing. It is critically important to word your request as a thank you for what is already done. Why? Because there is no present, no future. Time is a man-made construct. Einstein proved this. Everything is happening in the now. Somewhere in the now your problem has been solved and you are thanking the Universal Presence for the solution. IT IS ALREADY DONE!

Following are sections on developing a spa-like atmosphere in your home, and on meeting your guides.

Once comfortable, with your intentions clearly spoken, it is time to begin..

Chapter 6

YOUR HOME IS YOUR WELLNESS SPA

To concentrate on wellness in your life, you must consider how important the spaces in your life are. The space in which you live should be conducive to peace and healing. If you are attempting to lose weight, to regain control of your health and to bring your life to center, it becomes virtually impossible to do so in a chaotic, cluttered environment. A dirty home that is loud, with blaring TV's, with clutter and with confusion will not move you forward. Your home will get in the way of your progress.

I think of our home as our sanctuary, a safe place in which to do my work, both in meditation and in simply living my life. Your home reflects you and your life can reflect your home. How do you feel when you step into a spa? Most people instantly relax, with the calming sounds, smells, lighting and atmosphere. Imagine feeling this way when you walk through your front door! You can indeed.

A person with a cluttered mind will generally have a cluttered home. The clutter will get in the way of the flow of the vital energy required for a healthy life. Imagine the stagnant energy, dust, and who-knows-what lurking in corners of clutter. Energy will become stuck and stagnant there as well. For this reason, it's important to examine your living space with a critical eye towards peace and organization.

Look around you and take a deep breath. Can you visualize breathing clean air from every corner of every room in your home? If you cannot, then it would be helpful to begin to clear away the clutter and make some decisions as to priorities with your 'stuff'.

Of course, we can't all have spacious living spaces with room to spare. But as I found when we moved recently after living in the same place for fourteen years, there was a massive amount of 'stuff' - unidentifiable and unnecessary and it was taking up valuable living and breathing space in our home. It was indeed a big task, but we began to get rid of it. If it hadn't been used, seen or touched for years, then you won't miss it if you throw it out. Yard sales are an option. Charities are happy to take items for their thrift stores. This applies to every room in the house. I found that my kitchen was a real collector of unused culinary technologies, cookware, bakeware and utensils. If I'd not used it, I got rid of it.

The net benefit of this culling was a living space with BREATHING space as well. Suddenly my personal energy didn't feel stagnated any longer. I felt more relaxed. And of course, moving away from the hidden toxic black mold was a life saver for my husband, our fur and feather babies and myself.

While we don't all have the luxury of placing rooms and houses in particular angles with proper land alignment for optimum energy, Feng Sui is still of value for all spaces. The principles of Feng Sui will help you to identify stagnant areas, problem corners, areas that can be more 'free' and spaces that can benefit from a fresh eye.

Once the physical clutter of our living space was cleared, my meditation practice became far more progressive.

You may consider adding peaceful sounds to your home. I have a particular affinity for burbling water, and have numerous fountains in and surrounding our home. The cats have a gurgling water fountain, and I have a fountain outside our front door, and two on the patio. This flow of water is a constant reminder of peace.

We have placed Sonos speakers throughout our home and can use music services such as Pandora to channel spa music to any room at any time. I download music from iTunes or similar services and create nature playlists with bird songs and streams, or various types of relaxing music.

A peaceful home inspires all the senses. Obviously with less clutter, it is visually more relaxing. With water and music, it sounds more relaxing. And then there is the sense of smell. Adding light, unobtrusive healthy scents from aromatherapy oils can add another layer of peace to your home. Choose organic oils and diffuse a few drops into purified water using an ultrasonic diffuser to purify and lightly humidify the air in your home, creating a spa atmosphere.

Now, your clutter is cleared, your breathing is improved, your mind and heart are soothed by the atmosphere you've created and you are a step closer to healing your body. Your sleep should be improved, and of course, sleep is the key to any healthy lifestyle. This will all make it easier to clear the clutter and chatter from your active mind - theoretically.

For me, a peaceful space is the biggest requirement for a successful meditation practice.

Chapter 7

MEETING YOUR GUIDES

If you have done energy work before, then you know your spirit guides. You are always welcome to work with them and they welcome the opportunity to be of service to you. They are with you at all times, though you may not always hear them. However, if you do not know your guides, angels and spirit helpers, you may discover them in your meditations.

My guides made themselves known to me in meditations following my Reiki certification fourteen years ago. However, even before that, I always felt there was something or someone helping me. You may get a sense of their physical appearance. You might just get a sense of their energy or purpose. You will always get a sense of their love for you.

If you wish to learn more about your guides, you might consider working with an intuitive healer or energy worker for the sole purpose of contacting your guides and getting an understanding of how they wish to help you.

If you can come to know your spirit guides, it will help you immensely in your meditation practice as well as in your life in general.

Who are they? They are incorporeal beings that have been connected with us since before we are born. They often have been with us through many lives and incarnations. They help us daily, guide us through life and do their best to help us make the right decisions. Before we come into this life, there are contracts made with ourselves and with those who may incarnate with us in this lifetime. The guides help us while we're living this life.

Many guides stay with you throughout this lifetime, and some are more transient, coming and going as needed and to help with specific challenges and specific areas of your life, or to help with certain goals that you may have chosen to strive for. These guides have various talents and are at various levels of ascension and growth themselves. Some are very highly evolved, and others are just your 'average joe' of a spirit with talents in specific areas. They are essentially energy, but you may feel a male or female energy about them. Some have had physical form in the past. Some may have never taken a physical form. You could be their only 'project' and they guide only you. Or they could be working with others as well. But know this: When you need them, they will be there for you. They are in tune with you and will always be there when you ask for them. It is up to you, though, to try to listen for and to them, and to try to ascertain their guidance and the signs that they may send.

In my case, I'm very aware of my spirit guides who have been with me for many, many years and perhaps other lifetimes. Sometimes I sense additional guides - a new presence so to speak - to help with special goals and issues.

Once you are aware that you have spirit guides, then is the time for you to try to become sensitive to their direction and help. Be open to signs, synchronicities, and intuition. Start to pay attention to new people that may appear in your life, and any feelings you may have that they and you may have a purpose together. They could be there to help with a problem or challenge. I often wonder if my guides are not sometimes pushing me together with other charges of theirs, so that we may help each other. I do know one thing, though. There are very few accidents in my life. Things just appear to work out for a reason.

The signs are often there, but there are times that it is difficult to interpret them. Recently, after a particularly emotional visit to a close family friend, I seemed to be getting signs. I have always been particularly close to this couple and they were very much like my 'second parents'. They never had children and they were always my safe refuge when things in my life weren't going as I hoped. She recently died rather suddenly and we are trying to spend a lot of time with him now that she has gone. On the long ride home as my husband drove, I saw some miraculous cloud formations. I know these were messages to me. I asked in my meditations what it meant and it appears they were meant to tell me that my guides are there, that my guides, angels and others have a great deal of love for me, and that they're working with me through this time of grief and pain. One of the clouds appeared to be three angels in profile, side by side. I work with the same three archangels every day. Another was a perfect, massive image of a bird in flight. It looked very much like a sea gull or a dove. I felt love when I saw this formation. My reaction to these cloud formations was one of very profound emotion.

That same morning, I had awakened in our friends' home at 5 AM, with a voice in my left ear. I've never had any clear instance of clairaudience before. This was a female voice, sounding almost like my own, and it sounded scratchy as if it were on an old-time radio or on an old Victrola record. There seemed to be electronic interference. I turned over, thinking it was just some sort of tingling nerve on that side of my head. The voice then came to me in my right ear. The voice was simply saying numbers, and then repeating the numbers. I still have no idea what that meant, but I do believe that the significance will come to me. It is something I was meant to hear. However, there is no doubt in my mind that this is a sign for me. Interpretation? That's another challenge!

Our guides are responsible for our gut feelings. If you meet someone and you instinctively feel there is something that is not true about them, you should pay attention to your gut. It is usually a simple nudge from our guides saying "Watch out for this person." or "Don't trust this person." My experience has been that every time I overrule this gut instinct, I find later that it was a mistake to do so. Very often, something just doesn't seem to be in sync with what they say and the impressions I get from them in other ways.

Sometimes a gut feeling will trigger alarm or

caution and I feel it's especially important to pay attention to those feelings. Some years back, my husband was going to a family event of his in the middle of the country - America's heartland, so to speak. I couldn't go because of work. But I felt from the beginning that it was a very bad idea. The warnings had me in tears, and my gut literally hurt from worry about this trip.

You see, we eat a very specific, clean diet and we do so for a reason. We are both gluten intolerant. We neither one eat red meat nor dairy. We eat very minimal sugar, none of the 'chemical' sugars on the market and no processed foods because of the poisons in our foods these days. He was going to the middle of the country where they live on beef, wheat and where there is no real acknowledgement of the dangers in our food. The last thing I told him before he got on the plane was "Don't eat crap!" Well, perhaps I was a bit more descriptive than that.

He left on a Friday, flew home on a Monday evening. Tuesday he began to have sharp pains in his abdomen. The pains didn't go away. In asking about what he ate, it was clearly a very bad diet. There was a lot of meat, very few vegetables, tons of glutens. At this point, he still didn't understand the toxicity that glutens represent to over half of the population, and that it is more than just something unhealthy - it can be fatal. To some, a tiny amount can do as much damage as a large amount. It's the chemistry of it, not necessarily the volume. The pain got worse and worse. On a visit to the GP on Thursday, the x-ray indicated a blockage in his small intestine. The doctor prescribed some over the counter laxatives and softeners, to try to move this along. It didn't move. On Friday, the GP was closed for some unknown reason and my husband's pain got worse. He tried a colon irrigation with a specialist at that point but it did not help. Finally on Saturday after a second unsuccessful colon irrigation, a trip to the emergency room was unavoidable. The gas had backed up in his abdomen to the point that he honestly looked pregnant. The gas had placed so much pressure on his internal organs that his gall bladder had been smashed and stones went everywhere. The resulting surgery was a nightmare. The surgeon had said it would take two hours. It took seven. The surgeon made mistakes. The hospital stay was fifteen days. It took my husband almost two years to heal from that.

This is a rather long story, but it shows what happened when my gut feeling was ignored. Of course, my husband has free will and can do as he pleases. But that doesn't mean that my gut feelings should be ignored!

Always pay attention to intuitive feelings that you may have. Sometimes a thought appears to come from nowhere, but in reality, this could be important information from your guides. Don't try to ignore your intuitive thoughts and feelings. They're there for a reason and your guides rely on this to help you.

My guides are complete nudges. In my case, they want something for me a great deal, and in spite of my procrastination, denial or disorganization, they keep pushing me forward. Case in point: this book! They've been pushing me to do this for some time and I'd had every excuse in the world not to do it. My excuses: "I'm not a writer". "I don't have anything that anyone wants to read." Yet they are persistent and feel that it's important for me and for others. Lately, they seem to have been clearing blocks of time for me that I can devote to writing just as I realized that my experience with weight loss and wellness, through meditation is indeed something that others can benefit from. I find that not only do I believe in it, I very much want to help others by sharing my experiences.

So, you're thinking that this sounds wonderful but how do you connect with and develop a relationship with your guides directly?

I've already mentioned that a gifted energy worker or talented psychic can help you to connect with your guides. This person can help you to identify your guides and help to make the introduction. From there, you are free to develop this relationship on your own.

You can also open up your dreams to them. Before going to sleep, invite your guides to join you in your dreams and ask them to help you remember them upon awakening. Keep a pad and pencil by the bed so you can immediately write down your impressions, even before you open your eyes.

Another method is to sit quietly in a room or a garden or at the beach. Close your eyes and breathe. Ask your guides to join you. Ask them to identify themselves and then, simply listen. More than likely, the answers you feel are not coming from you, but from them. You can ask their names. Ask how they look. Ask how they are helping you. You can ask them for help and ask them how to proceed.

      There is one guarantee. You will feel their love and their willingness to work with you and to be there for you.

.

Chapter 8

BELIEVING

What you believe actually WILL happen. And to set this process in motion, you must see, hear, feel, taste and know that this belief is real and that you have already reached your goal(s).

Once your mind is tuned to your new reality of a thinner, healthier you, then it is just a matter of time before it happens. But in that time, you must continue to reinforce that reality and encourage your body to move towards that goal. This is where visualization and your belief system(s) come into play.

When I had my initial back injury and was in the intensive eight hour-a-day therapy program twenty-two years ago, I was exposed to extensive information on the mind-body connection. At that time, in 1993, it was somewhat revolutionary to find this kind of thinking in a main-stream physical therapy facility. I feel blessed to have been sent there and it truly was the first time I was exposed to what has turned out to be my path to wellness. At that time, PBS was featuring Bill Moyer's "Healing and the Mind" series. It explored the part the mind plays in your everyday wellness as well as in healing the body. The administrator of the facility, Dr. Andrew Rózsa, wholeheartedly embraced this thinking and shared the series with me and other patients. Inspired by his enthusiasm, I became a willing disciple. Dr. Rózsa is the first person that explained to me that the only person truly interested in my healing is going to be ME. He said that insurance companies, attorneys and doctors profit from my injuries and pain in many ways and that the best way to live a free life is to be free of them all. I took his lessons to heart and feel blessed to have learned from him.

It is important to use all of your senses to create your new reality of wellness and health. Thus, you can close your eyes and SEE your thin, healthy body. You can feel your body shrink, the fat disappear and can feel the new energy and vitality take the place of the sluggish old you. You can smell the air around your body and around your healthy life. You can breathe more easily without the extra weight draining your energy. You can hear the reactions to your glowing health from those you meet every day. You actually crave healthy foods and taste the foods that will make a dramatic difference in your vibrant health and in your wellness.

See the clothing that you wear once you're not encumbered by those extra pounds. See yourself moving more easily and going about your day with less strain on your body, thanks to the missing pounds that were putting stress on your joints and causing unnecessary pain. Your body wasn't meant to deal with this extra weight and without it, you're far more free to move . Imagine yourself with unlimited energy, a bright outlook on life and on your future. Feel the smile on your face when dealing with the people in your life, the new joy of living in this plane of existence. Enjoy the pep in your step, the new-found interest in the small things in life and the everyday miracles that surround you. For me, once the weight began to fall off, my world brightened, my attitude brightened and my mind became more engaged in all that surrounded me.

Colors were brighter. Smells more pronounced. The sense of touch was enhanced as was the sense of sound and taste. Yes, this is the result of meditation and the resulting weight loss. The entire experience has given me a far more positive outlook on everyday life, as well as an optimism that I had always wished would come more easily to me.

From this moment, begin to see yourself as thinner, brighter, happier, more positive, more active and see yourself involved in life at an entirely different level than before.

Leave behind the negative thinking. No more 'I can't'. Those words and thoughts do not serve you in your new reality. It's time to leave the past behind. Leave the pain behind. Live in the now and know that this exact moment is the only moment you are truly guaranteed. If you live this moment authentically, then any moments that follow will exponentially increase your spiritual and physical growth.

In meditation as in your life, being in the NOW is the key. Thus you must truly believe that you already have accomplished your goals and you must truly KNOW that your success is complete. Thank those guides, friends, spirits, angels, archangels, ascended masters and others who have helped you with your success every chance you get. It is rewarding for them to know that you have grown thanks to their help and that you acknowledge their part in your growth.

Chapter 9

VISUALIZATION, IMAGERY AND AFFIRMATIONS

Visualization is an important part of all of my meditations, be it for weight loss, healing or other issues or joys in my life. Breathing deeply will start the process of relaxation and will help you to find your center. But the key to success in my case has been visualization. I'm a firm believer: What you see will happen. What you believe to be true IS true.

This is actually very similar to a technique I used thirty five years ago when teaching others how to train their employees. The basis of the technique was the simple phrase "I see, I hear, I do, I understand". The more senses one uses to learn, the more ingrained the new reality will become. I see my new reality in my meditations. I experience what is happening to my body and what is happening around me.

I will share my visualizations techniques, but you are free to design your own. You should do what feels right for you.

Visualizing the fruits of your hard work and seeing

your success become a reality is a joyful experience.

It is necessary at times, to do some research in advance so that you can have a realistic basis for your visualization and imagery. This is, of course, my preference and you could also go more 'free form' with this. Since I am working on my body's systems, I personally prefer to have a somewhat realistic view of my body and how it works. You can get a clear roadmap of your body's organs and placement by Googling "organs of the body". I know we all saw these depictions as students in biology, but sometimes it doesn't hurt to jog the memory. This will give you an image to use in your meditation as a healthy depiction of your body.

With this basic knowledge, you can now become creative with your visualization. Use whatever you feel is helpful to you to encourage your body to operate properly and in a healthy manner.

As an example, I use an image of my thyroid gland. It is the largest gland in the neck area. A butterfly shaped organ that wraps the trachea, the sole function of this gland is to make the thyroid hormone. This may seem to be somewhat minor but the truth is that the thyroid hormone has an effect on almost all functions in the body. This gland's function is to regulate the body's metabolism. Because of the massive number of toxins that we encounter on a daily basis, the thyroid gland has been under attack for at least 70 years thanks to the introduction of fluoride to public water supplies. Municipalities have been duped into adding this toxic by-product of aluminum production to water supplies, under the guise of it's health benefits. The fact is that fluoride can completely shut down the thyroid gland and other important parts of your body or cause malfunction of this and other glands. For this reason, we have eliminated all the fluoride that we possibly can from our diets and our home. We use fluoride-free toothpaste and mouth rinses, and filter our water to remove fluoride among other contaminants. And remember, breathing fluoride and chlorine steam in the shower is every bit as toxic as drinking these contaminants. Your skin, the largest organ of your body, will absorb these chemicals from bath water and your shower. We filter our shower and bath water for fluoride and other metals.

    I begin my visualization with the image of my body as it should be - trim, healthy, disease free, active and pain free.   As I progress, I ask for healing for my body and work through the organs of my body that I feel I need help with. In my case, I am often remiss when it comes to drinking enough water during the day. So I have a specific visualization for my kidneys as vibrant and working properly. My visualization for my healthy, properly-functioning thyroid is in every meditation, every day. While the true symbiotic relationship between the thyroid gland, hypothalamus and pituitary gland is somewhat complicated, for the purpose of my meditation visualization, I simplify it so that I can visualize the benefit of a properly functioning thyroid gland.

Part of visualization for me involves feeling the changes in my body. For example, I visualize the thyroid hormone being produced as a neon blue charged fluid, and pumped throughout my body and my now-active metabolism begins to deal with the excess fat in my body. I imagine the unneeded fat globules in my body disintegrating and exiting through my pores, being gathered and sent to the ethers for recycling. And then I ask my body to tighten the skin behind the exiting fat cells. I feel the skin tighten from my toes to the top of my head. I see the trim, active, healthy me.

If you have health issues that have affected your weight, this is a good time to address them as well. In my case, my damaged back and joints has affected my ability to move as I would like, and so in my meditation, I visualize healing for my spine, hips, joints and any other area that requires healing.

You may visualize as a glowing, warm light that stimulates healing. You might visualize tiny medical avatars or fairies that work on your injuries to heal you. In my case, I combine many modalities in my healing visualization.

I prefer to work with colors which correlate with crystals. Since I use crystals in my meditation that correspond with various chakra centers, I often use these colors in my visualizations and imagery. I also work with angels and guides who have specific purposes and skills and who are always happy to be asked to be of service.

So prepare for your visualizations. In the section on meditation, I will detail my visualizations. Remember, these are the visualizations that resonate for me. You might find you can develop your own visualizations and imagery that will work for you.

When seeking growth and control of your body and your wellness, affirmations are invaluable. As discussed previously, what you believe will happen. Inserting positive affirmations during your day is a powerful way to train your mind to not only concentrate on your goals, but to eliminate negative thinking.

Write down your affirmations, insert them into your meditation but also, I put them on sticky notes where I'll think of them and repeat them all during my day. I put them on my computer screen, my bathroom mirror, in the kitchen where I work and near the fax machine and credit card machines in my office.

These affirmations might be:

* I am a powerful, healthy, thin person.
* I weigh a healthy ___ pounds
* My body functions optimally

* My thyroid is active and my body burns fat efficiently.
* My body utilizes nutrients efficiently

* I am blessed with abundant health, love, and gifts in my life
* I receive miracles every day

Create your own. The list can be long. When you repeat these to yourself all day long, you will find that your mind and body accepts these as truth and your body will begin to comply.

Chapter 10

MEDITATIONS

To start, be sure that you have everything at hand that you might need. Many people are able to meditate successfully without the following, but with our busy lives and active minds, most of us need all the help we can get to let go of the daily stresses and worries, the mundane thoughts that will wander in and out of your consciousness, and to relax to do this work.

If you are unsure of the basics of meditation and are looking for a quick start of sorts, my friend Elissa Bentsen has contributed her quick steps to meditation, which you will find in Appendix IV "Quick Start to Meditation."

Let's review the list:

<u>An appropriate space</u> By now, you should have identified the appropriate space in your home for this work. Be sure you will not be interrupted by external noises, phone calls or pets. It's time to turn it all off because this time is for you. If you plan to use aromatherapy, prepare your diffuser and turn it on. If you plan to use aromatherapy sprays, then lightly spray in the area where you will be working as well as over your head, repeating and concentrating on the intention you wish to

accomplish. For instance, if you're using an Archangel Raphael spray, spritz lightly over your head and in the area where you will sit or lie, and say "I thank you, Archangel Raphael, for my successful weight loss and achieving my wellness goals".

<u>Know the spirit guides and angels that you may wish to call upon:</u> These helpers will give you strength, ideas and support in all that you wish to accomplish.

<u>Any other aids or crystals:</u> If you wish to use crystals, then have them close at hand. I prefer to use crystals on my chakra points and thus, to place the crystals, I find that I need to lie down. Those pesky stones just won't stay put on my heart chakra if I'm sitting up!

<u>Music or ambient sounds:</u> If you wish to use music or ambient sounds, have your iPhone, iPod or other audio device set with the track(s) you wish to use. Have your ear buds or headphones comfortably in place. To keep an eye on the time for your meditation, then you'll want to know how long each track is. Set your tracks to repeat if you wish. Many days I'd love to just go on and on with my meditation but life is always waiting. In my case, my preferred sound track is about a half-hour long, so I set it on repeat. If I have allotted an hour for my meditation, then I know when it has repeated twice, that I'm at my limit and it's time to wrap it up. If I have more time, then I can judge appropriately.

<u>Prepare for your visualizations</u>: You should research in order to have the proper visualizations at your

mental fingertips as you progress in your meditation.

<u>Situate yourself comfortably:</u> If you are sitting, sit comfortably with both feet planted on the ground, spine and neck straight. If you choose to lie down, then be sure that your spine is straight, that your body is in alignment and you are comfortable. Remember, you may be in this position for an hour or so. With my back injuries, I place a pillow under my knees to take the strain off of my lower back. If you're using crystals, place the appropriate crystals in the appropriate chakra area. This is a good way to draw your concentration to the energy centers in your body. If you are sitting, you may place the crystals in your palm that you feel will be helpful in your session. Cover yourself lightly if you feel it will make you more comfortable. Allow your arms to lie by your side, or slightly extended from your shoulders flat beside if you're lying flat. If you're sitting, allow your arms to hang comfortably from your shoulders by your side, palms up, hands opened naturally and comfortably.

<u>Start your music or sounds.</u> Adjust the volume.

<u>Breathe deeply</u> A Prana style of breathing is recommended, with your tongue against the top of your mouth and the tip of your tongue just behind your upper front teeth. Start with three deep breaths. Breathe in through your nose, allowing the air to completely fill your lungs, first filling the bottom of your lungs, and then to the top. This process should take about seven seconds. Allow the breath to linger there about four seconds, and then, breathe out through your mouth, totally emptying the

lungs from the top, to the bottom, pushing the air out as much as possible for about seven seconds. Repeat at least three times. If you find you're distracted, then continue the breathing until it is the only thought in your mind.

With each breath, feel your body relax and feel yourself go more deeply into a state of blissful relaxation. Mentally work your way to your extremities, allowing each breath to deeply relax the muscles in your core, your back, your upper legs, your knees, your calves, your ankles and your feet. Allow your legs and feet to feel heavy. Imagine your palms and feet feeling warm. Imagine the warmth flowing up your arms and legs to your core. Continue allowing the breath to relax the shoulders, upper arms, lower arms, wrists and hands. Now feel the breath relax your neck and jaw. Feel the muscles of your face relax. Notice that your scalp is relaxed and that your head is resting comfortably on the pillow if lying down. If sitting, your head is perfectly balanced on your spine.

<u>Your first visualization</u>: Imagine that you are in a place that is peaceful and comfortable for you. This could be a beautiful garden with lush planting, flowers, birds and wildlife. It could be by the sea, with your feet in the sand. It could be on a mountain top or cliff, overlooking a beautiful valley or overlooking the ocean. You choose the place. Now, visualize the earth and how it was formed, and how this place came to be. Think of the power of the original earths' core, the heat and lava that formed the rock. Think of the winds and rains that wore the rock down and created the soil, which became the home of seeds. These seeds grew, enriched by our sun, the rains

and the minerals in the soil. This is the place where you live. You are a product of this beautiful planet and you should feel the energy and joy that this planet represents.

<u>Grounding</u> Any type of meditation or energy work requires grounding and protection. Now that you are in a beautiful place, and you are part of this amazing planet, visualize your root chakra at the base of your spine and with a mighty exhale, extend a cord or a trunk from the base of your spine into the earth. I visualize a tree trunk in a rich red color which is the color for your root chakra. I see it go deep into the earth, grounding me and spreading roots much like a tree, taking in the energies from the planet.

Then I visualize energy from the earth being drawn from the roots with my inhale and through the trunk, through me, as a column of light extending up through my open crown into the heavens. I breathe the earth energy in, and breath it out into the heavens allowing it to begin flowing on its' own. I repeat this until it begins to feel automatic. Then, I visualize energy from the heavens flowing down through my crown, into the earth. With every inhale, I breathe in the light from the heavens. With every exhale, I send that energy into the earth until it becomes automatic.

At this point, the energy begins flowing both ways, through me and I am a conduit between heaven and earth, and encased in the column of light.

<u>Protection:</u> Now is the time to ask for protection.

During this work, you can be vulnerable to energies that may not be benevolent, so protection is important. One of my guides has always provided me with peace and love and protection in my home. I visualize lying my head on her lap on her silky skirt, and I feel comforted in that moment, asking for a safe, protected bubble around us in which we can do our work. I ask that only the angels, guides and entities with the highest purpose be allowed in our space, or anyone who I may invite into the space. I imagine this space to be a soft rose color, since this is the color I associate with my guide. I then also ask Archangel Michael to put an extra protective shield around our bubble. (For this exterior shield, I use an electric blue image.) Allow a time to settle in to this bubble and to luxuriate in its safety, breathing deeply the entire time.

All the while I'm part of the light and energy from the heavens and from the earth that is flowing through me and through the space.

<u>Fill your bubble with love:</u> You've created a safe space to do your work. It's important to now come from a place of love and to fill this space with love. There are many ways to do this and it will eventually become a very specific and personal step for you.

I begin by sending love to a few persons who are now on the other side. For me, it is easy to tap into the immense love for my mother, my maternal grandmother and a very dear friend and to send it to them. When you send love, you will get it back a thousand fold. For me, the love and emotion is overwhelming. The love that is sent back begins to fill the space. Be sure you're still breathing deeply and breathe this love in and breathe it out of your heart chakra, until your entire body is filled with love.

Then I send love to my spirit guides. I invoke each by name and send them love and massive gratitude for the miracles that happen every day in my life thanks to them. They each have their specialties and I thank them specifically for the manner in which they've each enriched my life. I feel their love wrapping around me, and flowing through my heart, front to back and back to front, intersecting with the column of light from the heavens and the earth.

Then I send love to my archangels, angels, and other spirits. By now the bubble is packed with love!

This is the time that I listen for messages from my loved ones on the other side and when I can share messages with them. You should be feeling very peaceful and loved at this point, breathing in the love and breathing it out.

This is when I begin my meditation for health and wellness. I always repeat my requests and my gratitude three times, in great detail.

<u>Defining my weight goal</u>: I begin by expressing my gratitude to Archangel Raphael and all of my guides and helpers that I am now a healthy ____ pounds, pain free, disease-free and active. I thank them profusely for

my healthy, vibrant, disease-free mind, body, spirit and heart that are tied together in longevity. (After all, we don't want our body nor our minds to outlast the other parts, do we?) I express my gratitude from the heart with great love. I repeat this three times, breathing deeply as I continue to express my gratitude.

Remember, 'time' in the angelic and non-earth realms is different than our time, and there is little if any distinction between now and the future. In those realms, everything is as it is. Thus it is important to always think in the now, not in the future or the past. What you ask for has happened or is happening now. Thus try to remain in the present during this process.

A: Meditation for General wellness and "Massage Method":

I have three separate but similar methods that I've used for weight loss and general wellness. The first one, the 'massage method' is what I used initially while training my body to release the unnecessary fat. After I became adept at this, I was able to alter this visualization to concentrate on general wellness.

I begin by expressing my gratitude for Archangel Raphael and the medical avatars for healing my body in any and all areas that need healing. The color surrounding Archangel Raphael is green, thus you can always evoke that color for all healing in your body and in your life. I envision the avatars as healing beings and generally green, who can be very small when necessary or very large as required, for physical healing. I then ask that the medical avatars begin to work the unnecessary fat cells loose in my body so that they may be recycled into the ethers. Essentially, I go through an entire full-body massage in my mind with this.

I start imagining a moderate massage starting with my feet, working up through the ankles and paying attention to any swelling or fatty areas there. Since most massage modalities entail movement from the extremities towards the heart, I use this. I imagine the massage continuing up my calves to my knees and again, paying special attention to any swelling, painful or fatty areas there. The massage continues through my body, over my thighs, front and back, and then to my hips, buttocks and abdomen. In my case, the thighs, hips, buttocks and abdomen need special attention. Once I feel that area has been thoroughly worked over, I continue with the mental massage up my sides, in my back through shoulders and neck.

The massage continues from my hands, working up from my fingers, to my wrists, forearms, upper arms and shoulders, to my chest and neck. Then I enjoy to a facial and cranial massage.

The entire time, with every massage stroke, I visualize miniscule globules of fat coming through my skin, gathering just outside my bubble in a big blob that to me, looks like the disgusting fat that comes from meats in the grocery store. Once the blob is suitably large, I dispatch it for recycling. After all, there are animals and people on the planet who don't have enough to eat and enough body fat to maintain them. I prefer to think that I've helped them in some way. Again, this is just a thought and visualization that I use to move the fat from me, hoping it will do someone some good elsewhere.

Now, I breathe deeply, feeling lighter and thinner. I imagine the skin tightening where there had been the excess fat. If it feels right, I try to enjoy this sensation of overall tingling, tightening and smoothing of my body.

Now I begin to work on the inside. In my research, I found images of fat that has gathered inside the body, surrounding organs in the abdominal cavity so I begin to concentrate on that in the same manner that I have dispatched the other fatty deposits. It flies away, for recycling!

I ask that my spine be healed, and use imagery of the tiny, medical avatars working to repair my disks, ruptures, herniations and other spinal injuries, restoring health to the spinal cord and to all that connects to it. I ask that these small miracle workers stay with me as long as is necessary during the day to continue to repair my spine and other joint injuries.

I again ask Archangel Raphael for healing, and begin to visualize my internal organs at their peak performance. While I know this is not how the kidneys might visually work, I do give them a mental boost at this time, imagining that they work as a centrifuge of sorts, sending rich, clean blood to the body and sending waste and urine products for elimination. I imagine my colon is clean and working properly, that my liver is working properly and that it, along with my gall bladder, are eliminating fats. I imagine a properly functioning stomach and digestive tract. I imagine my heart pumping properly, with no fat around it, and I imagine that my veins and arteries are free of clogs and flexible. I visualize healthy, pink lungs and imagine that they are being scrubbed of toxins or remnants of second hand cigarette smoke that I've been unable to avoid.

Now I move up to my thyroid, visualizing it as an electric blue butterfly, working with the pituitary gland and hypothalamus to send electric blue impulses through my body, burning unnecessary bits fat that I've been unable to dispatch thus far. I imagine this continuing all through the day.

I imagine my brain is vibrant, disease free with no tau, no plaque and nothing that would hamper my ability to think, reason and remember. I ask that the medical avatars eliminate any impediments they find to clear thinking, active brain function and a clear memory.

I thank Archangel Raphael for the amazing healing and show my emotional gratitude for the daily miracles that I receive.

B: General wellness and visualization "Glowing

Wellness method":

After I used the above method for several months and as the weight began to drop, I began to modify my meditation specifics somewhat. I still use the above once a week, but now I often use an altered version, as detailed below.

This visualization is similar but concentrates on glowing wellness as well as weight loss.

After expressing gratitude for my desired weight, I again ask for healing. I feel warmth at my extremities, moving to the center of my body, and feel all organs of my body, operate in sync. I imagine my skeletal frame and joints moving smoothly with the ligaments, tendons and other soft and connective tissue doing their jobs. The warmth represents healing. I feel my body is in sync.

I imagine the warmth pushing any unwanted fat through my pores, out of my body and into the area above my safe bubble, where it is sent for recycling.

Again, from the outer extremities, I begin to feel relaxation, with all tension letting go from my toes and finger tips, to the center of my body. My neck relaxes. My shoulders relax. I float and yet feel totally supported, and relaxed, breathing in the love that surrounds me.

C: The Winds wellness and visualization method:

This third method of course, uses all the same

techniques as in the previous methods. I express gratitude for my current healthy weight of ____ (your goal) and that I am pain-free. I thank Archangel Raphael for my healthy, vibrant, disease-free mind, body, spirit and heart that are tied together in longevity. I express this gratitude three times, and at all times, my heart is bursting with love and thanks.

As I breathe deeply, I imagine that my breath is a soothing wind entering my body from my core with every inhale. The wind is refreshing and invigorating. I direct the healing wind first down my legs, to my toes, my feet, my ankles and feel it swirling, releasing any remaining pain, discomfort and any fat that may be there. I feel the wind blowing towards my knees, my thighs and my hips, always swirling, always cleansing and always breathing new life into each part of my body as it circles back to my core with each exhale.

Next I imagine the wind down my arms, to my finger tips, hands, wrists, elbows and shoulders, again, releasing pain with each swirl. I see the discomfort and any body fat that is there now leaving that area, and traveling with the wind towards my core.

Now the wind is swirling throughout my entire body, and in doing so, it pushes unwanted fat out of my body, into the area above my safe bubble, where it is sent for recycling.

I then release the pain, the discomfort, the fat and any disease that may be in the wind.

Again, the wind enters my body with every inhale, this time working through my internal organs, from my colon all the way up to my shoulders, up my spine, again releasing and clearing any pain, disease and fat. It is then released from my body with every exhale.

The wind continues again, up through my shoulders and neck, releasing any tension and pain. The swirling wind enters my head, clearing any fears and any disease.

With every breath, I feel healed and loved.

I thank Archangel Raphael for all of his help with my ability to meditate easily and comfortably and to accomplish my goals. I also thank him for the growth of my clairvoyant, clairsentient and clairaudient gifts. I thank my guide who works with Archangel Raphael and gives me daily guidance in the form of crystal energies, natural remedies and suggestions for myself, my husband and my pets.

Gratitude is the biggest part of the entire process. (see Appendix V: Gratitude Exercise) Remember, all of this happens in the now and not in the past, not in the future. Thus you have every reason to thank your guides and angels for the joys and miracles in your life and, of course, YOU and your wellness and weight loss are just one of the many miracles you are experiencing.

Once you feel totally, completely relaxed, this is a

good time to simply 'be', immersed in gratitude and love, and listen. Breathe in the air of healing around you, and breathe out any unwanted fats, toxins and illness that may have been in your body. Breathe in wellness. Breathe out pain. Concentrate on your body's new thin feel. Notice that your arms are thin, your legs are thin, your waist and buttocks are thin and your stomach and abdomen are flat. Enjoy the feeling of freedom that you feel without the burdensome weight that you've been carrying around. The weight put pressure on your joints, on your back, on your life. The weight is now gone so it no longer encumbers you.

Notice how light you are on your feet now, and how every step is a joy, not a burden.

This is the new 'set point' for your body. If you continue to feel this in meditation and your body believes that it is so, it WILL be so. If you do not allow negative thoughts, your body will have no reason to react negatively.

Listen for any instructions or ideas that our guides have for your wellness and your weight-loss regimen. Thoughts may come to you and you wonder if they are your thoughts or if they are from your guides. If they feel as if they are new ideas, new concepts, then more than likely they are coming from your guides. If they feel as if they are an intrusion from the 'real world', then it is possible that these thoughts are yours and a bit of your 'monkey brain' chatter. Acknowledge these intrusive thoughts, and firmly blow them aside, knowing you can address them later in the day.

This is when I have the greatest revelations concerning issues with my body that may need to be addressed. Languish in this state as long as you wish.

I now move on to Archangel Michael. Archangel Michael is the ultimate go-to angel when it comes to protection and simply making things happen. I see his presence often during my day. I ask for his help when there is an electronic or mechanical malfunction. If you find you're seeing a bright, neon blue or bright, neon purple, you know that Archangel Michael is there. I might see it repeated several times in the shirt colors people are wearing, or in signs. I thank Archangel Michael for his protection of my health, my home and my loved ones, picturing each in a protective, bright blue bubble. I thank Archangel Michael for protecting our electronics, our furniture and belongings, our finances, and our vehicles. I thank him for keeping our vehicles and electronics working properly. I thank him for protection when we are traveling in our vehicles, whether short trips or long trips. Every time I go to my car, I ask Archangel Michael for protection and safety.

Archangel Michael is also the angel to ask for emergency help. If you have an emergency medical issue for yourself or even an emergency mechanical or electrical issue, ask Archangel Michael to help. Ask him for help three times "Help me, Archangel Michael." Then three times, thank him for his help in solving the specific emergency issue.

Now breathe in Archangel Michael's brilliant energy and listen for any messages he may have for you.

From this point, you may wish to access other angels and guides. When you set your intentions for your meditation session, you should have an idea of what you hope to accomplish and should know which angel or guide is best able to help you.

Once I have consulted with other guides and angels, and am feeling at peace, I then thank each guide and each angel individually for their help, and express the gratitude for the love in my life, the people in my life and the miracles that surround me every single day.

I open my eyes slowly, breathe deeply, and enjoy the moment.

After my daily meditation, I enjoy a glass of water, and take my time moving into my day, moving slowly, breathing deeply, and I make it a point to appreciate all that surrounds me at that moment, and the beauty of the day.

Chapter 11

PUTTING IT ALL TOGETHER

Please remember that the purpose of my book is not to tell anyone how to take care of their own health, wellness and how to manage their weight. This is the story of my journey and my growth from this journey. It is my sincere hope that you will be inspired by my discoveries, both medical and spiritual, and create your own journey to health, weight loss, wellness and personal growth.

You can choose foods that are nutritious, healthy, supportive and that will give you the energy and support that your body needs. I urge you to select organic and non-GMO foods.

You can eliminate toxins from your home, your body and your work environment.

You can begin an exercise or movement program that will help your body to burn calories and unnecessary fat.

If you're not seeing results, then I encourage you to seek the help of an integrated medical professional to find the road blocks that are more than likely stunting your results. Evaluate your environment and water seeking any possible contaminants and toxins that are blocking progress. Read all labels of anything that you consume.

You can order some tests yourself in your quest to address issues that could be blocking your progress. The ALCAT can be ordered online and they will send a tech to your home for the blood draw if there is not an authorized testing center near you. You can also order blood tests from Life Extension without having to start with a doctor, should you so prefer. Please note, though, that your health insurance will probably not cover these tests if not ordered by a doctor.

Once this has all been addressed, if you're still not dropping pounds, meditation is going to be the final step.

Even if you have noticed significant improvement, I still recommend meditation. It will make a difference in the quality of your life and your ability to maintain your weight loss.

Be sure to fill your network with those who can and will support your journey and your thinking. Don't allow negativity to take hold EVER!

You are now in control of your body, your wellness, your weight and your life.

APPENDIX I: CHOLESTEROL

Don't be sidetracked by the usual demons found in blood tests. You could lose valuable time and effort, and even add further toxins to your body following some of the myths peddled by our current standard medical community. One of the big demons? Cholesterol!

Initially, my cholesterol numbers were high - in the 240 total cholesterol range - so I cut out almost anything with meaningful cholesterol. The cholesterol went down somewhat but is still not in the medically defined 'normal' range. However, since then, I've done some in-depth study on my own of cholesterol and it's function in the body. An astounding fact became evident: Even with all the research done since the 1950's, dietary cholesterol and high blood cholesterol numbers have never been SHOWN to cause heart disease, stroke or other conditions commonly used as scare tactics when doctors discuss your cholesterol. There is no evidence that high cholesterol levels CAUSE heart disease. As it happens, this thinking came about by simple association. One may have high cholesterol and may have heart disease, but there is no proof that cholesterol CAUSES heart disease. Add to that the billion dollar pharmaceutical companies' never-ending push to doctors to sell their statin drugs, and doctors who choose the 'easy way' to deal with the demonized cholesterol obsession by simply writing a script and you end up with the cholesterol obsession that has plagued our society for the 28 years since statins were introduced on the market. Had I taken statin drugs, my problems and symptoms would have multiplied. Some side effects include headache, sleeplessness, muscle aches, increased liver enzymes, tenderness, inflammation of the muscles and severe muscle damage. Sadly, this is one of the most prescribed drugs in this country, right along with antacids and proton pump inhibitor drugs. These drugs, by the way, do a great deal of damage to the gastrointestinal tract and thus, inhibit your ability to absorb vital nutrients.

Continuing research shows that the association between cholesterol and heart disease and heart attacks has become a very weak claim. The truth is, your body NEEDS cholesterol. It is the lubricant that keeps the machine running! It is truly a building block for our body. It is part of the cell membrane of every cell in our body and without it your cells don't function properly. People with low cholesterol numbers are at risk for depression, suicide and psychosis and actually, the number of people who die of heart attack are 1 1/2 times more likely to have LOW cholesterol numbers. Cholesterol is necessary for your body to build and maintain important hormones such as testosterone, DHEA, estrogen and progesterone.

Like everything else in life, however, moderation is the key.

APPENDIX II: HORMONES

I read Suzanne Somers books concerning her journey with hormone therapy and the Wiley Protocol. While she's been actively and aggressively criticized by the western medical community, I read with great interest her findings and her results. I didn't find her to be a nut. I found her to be a profoundly earnest woman who did her homework and thought logically.

I also read the work of T.S. Wiley. Ms. Wiley's approach is far different than you'll find in the standard Western medical establishment. Her protocol uses compounded natural bioidentical hormone creams that are applied in a rhythmic, cyclic method., mimicking the human body's natural hormone cycles. Since her compounds are not made from chemicals nor from pregnant mares urine (i.e., Premarin) or other things that the Big Pharma drug companies use, they were more complimentary to the body's natural functions. The severely flawed, non-balanced, discontinued NIH study had become the mainstay of the medical community's direction in the field of hormone replacement therapy. The mainstream medical practitioners (mostly male) seemed unable to see the flawed methodology behind the failed NIH study and stubbornly refused to think beyond that in their fear-filled world.

As with all things pertaining to your health, balance is the key and there was absolutely no balance in the NIH study. Both progesterone and estrodial need to be working in harmony when using hormone therapy and the NIH study ignored that. Plus, their main ingredient was not natural, unless you consider pregnant mares' urine that's been chemically altered in a laboratory to be 'natural'.

As a lifelong non-smoker, and a woman who had not been on birth control for 18 years, there seemed no need for worry of risk factors. The trick was finding the right person to help me with hormones. Living in an area that might as well be a third world country when it comes to medical choices, this was a challenge. I made an appointment with a doctor in South Miami who had advertised the Wiley Protocol and told me they did it, then when I arrived, they tried to 'switch' me to something else. Obviously he was not the certified Wiley provider that he'd represented himself to be. His required, very expensive saliva testing proved to be useless - a mere snapshot of a day in a cycle that was not defined. And his scripts were oral and thus, going through the digestive tract and ineffective.

So there was yet another trip to the Miami area, this time to Aventura, to another practitioner. I found him to be a fascinating person and I liked his 'out of the box' thinking. He did indeed do the Wiley Protocol but his connection with compounding pharmacies was rather thin. I was on it a few months with good results, when the compounding pharmacy seemed to disappear. SO, I went forward with my search.

My husband had seen my improvement and had been reading about Wiley for men and wanted to try the Wiley Protocol for Men himself. We eventually found an integrative health care provider in Southwest Florida. Per the protocol, the proper testing was done and we were on the protocol with a reputable compounding pharmacy. We now blood test on the proper days of our cycle at least once a year to be sure our levels are where they are supposed to be. She adjusts as necessary for optimal results.

My husband swears he feels better and than he felt when he was 24. For me there is no foggy thinking, no hot flashes and no sleep issues. And miracles of miracles! This practitioner set us on the path of total wellness. She was the integrated medical practitioner that at the time, we didn't realize we needed.

So, that was the first step in the process. Once the hormones are functioning properly, then we began to do more comprehensive blood testing for other issues: Blood pressure, cholesterol, and much, much more.

As always, I recommend that you do your own research. You can find more about the Wiley Protocol and determine if it is right for you by going to their website at **www.TheWileyProtocol.com**. When you are researching this, you will find some negative articles about Ms. Wiley but, it seems, these are pretty much the bitter aftermath of a legal dispute between Ms. Wiley and her ex-business partner. Sadly, we all have to wade through this type of bad energy in doing any sort of research for our own wellness..

APPENDIX III: INJECTABLE AND LIPOSOMAL SUPPLEMENTS

Supplementation has been invaluable to our good health and to our future wellness, since our foods are sorely lacking in the nutrition that we all need. In many cases, oral supplementation is adequate. For some vitamins and nutrients, however, alternative delivery systems are necessary. Injectable and liposomal supplements have proven to be truly beneficial to us. The issue with oral supplements is that your digestive tract will effectively eliminate up to 98% of the benefit that you would expect to get from a supplement. For instance, you might take a 1,000 mg vitamin C capsule, thinking that you will get the benefit of 1,000 mg. However, the truth is that you'll be lucky to get 20 mg once your digestive tract and your stomach acids have finished with it. While there are many manufactured liposomal supplements out there, I have found the two that are most beneficial to us are Vitamin C and Glutathione. Vitamin C is a DNA protector and has proven important to protect workers exposed to severe radiation from free radical damage. It also helps manufacture collagen, which is necessary for the health of our tissues, teeth, joints and bones, repairs blood vessels and is important to normalize blood pressure. Vitamin C has been known to heal degenerative diseases and is an important weapon in the anti-aging battle. AND it helps keep your mood and outlook a happy one.

Dr. Linus Pauling, Nobel Prize winner, pioneered the concept of megadose vitamin therapy for those with serious illnesses. It is used today for anti-cancer treatments.

SO, knowing how important this vitamin is, as well as the B vitamins and glutathione, the best way to assure that you're getting the full benefit of important nutrients is to put them into your body tissues and blood stream directly. Vitamin B-12 injections are common as are injections for other vitamins. With this, you will get the full benefit of what is injected, and effectively saturating the body with the vitamin that your body requires. Your wellness provider will still need to write a prescription for these vitamins, though.

The FDA has made it more and more difficult for knowledgeable, ethical wellness practitioners and compounding pharmacies to bring us these supplements that are of such vital importance to all of us. You see, vitamins and natural substances cannot be patented, thus the Big Pharma companies are not willing to produce them. Unless it's been chemically altered in a lab, it cannot be patented and thus is open to the free market forces. Big Pharma doesn't want to do business on a level playing field and thus, they don't want to sell something where they would have actual, ethical competition.

The pharmaceutical companies are threatened by the sheer existence of these substances, as are the standard western medical community's practitioners who are not up to date on the value of these substances. Remember, vitamins and supplements fall into the category of nutrition and those with medical degrees get less than 20 hours of nutrition in their 8 years of medical school. It's a classic example of demonizing something that they simply do not understand. Add to that the fact that these medical people are unwilling to do the work to learn about alternative means of treatment and are heartily rewarded by their friends in Big Pharma to actively sell the drugs and pharmaceuticals with the myriad of dangerous side effects, and you can see where the vitriol towards wellness and supplementation is born.

There have been recent attacks on compounding pharmacies by the government, thanks to prodding by Big Pharma and the AMA. I strongly encourage all readers become involved in the effort to keep our compounded supplements available by contacting their lawmakers in Washington. It is important that we retain our right to choose for our own health and wellness, and that we have all the information available to us that we need to make these important decisions for ourselves. Much like labeling, it is important that your legislators know that you want to make these informed choices, and that they really should not take these options away from you by doing the bidding of the pharmaceutical companies as well as the AMA. You can find out more as well as a list of your legislators at **http://www.ProtectMyCompounds.com.**

You and your integrated wellness provider can work together to find the proper plan for you. And your informed provider can help develop formulas for your specific challenges, much as our provider has.

When I was ill two years ago, my wellness advisor, Mitzi Schardt, felt strongly that a series of IV pushes would be beneficial, but since she is six hours away from me, it was not something that we could easily accomplish. For instance, she felt that large doses of Vitamin C in an IV push would be helpful, as would large doses of glutathione in an IV push. But these two cannot be done on the same day and should be spaced apart and repeated for a period of time. So I did the initial glutathione push, but then learned to make my own in liposomal form.

The benefit of liposomals is that through the process (which is detailed below) the vitamin / nutrient is encased in nanoparticles, which protect the nutrient through the ravages of the digestive tract, allowing the nutrient to enter the body relatively intact, delivering at least 92% benefit.

Glutathione is essential to the body's ability to heal itself and to maintain vitality but oral supplementation is useless since the glutathione never makes it through the digestive system. The recommended effective dose of glutathione is around 440 mg daily. The glutathione recipe below delivers approximately that amount per 2 oz dose. The Vitamin C recipe below delivers around 1.688 gm per 2 oz. dose. For me, since they shouldn't be taken the same day, I double up alternating days, doing two doses of the Vitamin C on one day, and two doses of the glutathione the next.

What you need to make your liposomal supplements:

Ultrasonic cleaner: Since I'm making this for two

persons, I wanted a large, industrial grade machine that would hold up, and chose the Kendal Industrial Grade 165 watt, 2.5 liter Ultrasonic Cleaner. This should be around $89 from Amazon. You can buy elsewhere at varying prices. I find this to be an exceptional machine for the above use, and it's held up well for about a year and a half and is not showing signs of wear and tear in the least.

Sunflower Lecithin: Since this is the basis for entering directly into the cells of your body, I strongly recommend buying the best product possible. I've found that the Swanson Non-GMO Sunflower Lecithin has worked well for us, and I buy in 16 ounce container. If I could buy it in organic form, I would. As with many of my purchases, I use Amazon. We live in a town with few choices and shopping can be a nightmare. Avoid Soy Lecithin. Soy in all forms, except fermented, is a hormone disruptor and the last thing you need is putting something directly into your cells that can cause further damage to your body.

Vitamin C: There are many products available. Please feel free to shop but be sure you're getting something with equivalent nutrition. I use NOW Foods Vitamin C Crystals, ascorbic acid in a one pound container. The label on this product states that 1/2 tsp is 2.25 grams of Vitamin C / ascorbic acid. Using this number, I came up with the 1.688 GM number for a two ounce dose.

While there has been discussion about the differences in natural vitamin C and the ascorbic acid version of vitamin C, these are chemically identical. According to the Linus Pauling Institute, there have been no known differences in their biological activity, even though there have been several studies to determine what if any difference existed.

Reduced Glutathione: This is more difficult to find. Again, I went through Amazon. I've had good results with Bulk Supplements brand Pure Glutathione Reduced Powder in 100 gm packages.

Recipe for Liposomal Vitamin C

In a blender or Vitamix, add 6 level TBS of sunflower lecithin. Slightly warm 16 oz of purified water in a glass measuring cup. I warm it to the point where it feels to be around 98 degrees on my wrist, much like you do a baby's bottle. Add the 16 oz of warm water to the container of the blender. Process on high for a minute, until the mixture has a milky, beige look to it.

At the same time, warm another 16 oz of purified water in glass measuring cup. Add 2 level TBS of the Vitamin C. Stir with a wooden spoon. You may need to let this sit for five or ten minutes to allow the Vitamin C crystals to dissolve.

Into the clean ultrasonic machine, pour the lecithin mixture, and then the Vitamin C mixture. Stir with wooden spoon.

Process for a minimum of 4 cycles of 480 each. I try to process for at least 6 cycles, because the more times it is processed, the smaller the particles are and thus, more absorbable.

Store up to two weeks in the fridge. My husband takes this daily, so I pour this into two ounce 'jello shot' cups with lids, so he can easily grab one a day and drink up, without pouring and spilling. For me, since I alternate days, I grab two every other day.

Recipe for Liposomal Glutathione

This recipe will be identical to the above, except instead of dissolving Vitamin C into the second warmed 16 oz container of purified water, you will dissolve 2 TBS of the reduced glutathione.

You don't necessarily have to store this in jello shot cups. For this, since I take this and my husband does not, I just pour into a sterilized 32 oz glass jar and pour two - 2 oz servings every other day.

APPENDIX IV: QUICK START TO MEDITATION: 10 STEPS TO DEEP MEDITATION AND AWARENESS

This section is general information on meditation and the info below was contributed by Elissa Bentsen, founder of Forever Souls **www.ForeverSouls.com**, and a very gifted energy worker whom I have become friends with. She has helped me with soul healing and with solving problems in my life that surround past life trauma. However, her work as with all energy work, revolves around meditation. She has shared her simplified 10 steps to deep mediation, with her permission to published in this book. This information is a good 'quick start' for beginners to meditation. My meditation sessions generally last an hour, but it is difficult to control your mind's chatter for very long without practice. Indeed, as much as I mediate and as devoted as I am to daily meditation, there are days that I can't seem to quiet the monkey chatter in my head successfully for very long stretches. I simply acknowledge that it is, and try to move on.

Elissa's 10 steps are an excellent jumping off point to meditation. Some of her insights are below. From Elissa:

"The key to self-knowledge and opening to intuition is meditation. The Lightworker Guides with whom I communicate are insistent about daily meditation for any and all of life's challenges. Yet many people do not meditate and are unclear on how to begin a daily practice. To be clear, mediation takes practice. I remember Dr. Brian Weiss, once said it took him 30 days to achieve a deep meditative state.

Like any other good habit, it takes discipline and determination.

"If you Google "How to Meditate" you will find a zillion approaches, many are almost identical and some are extreme. Some suggest a time period of 15 minutes a day while others insist that anything under an hour is unproductive. In my experience, how long you mediate doesn't compare to how deep you go. 15 minute deep mediation can be more effective than a shallow one hour session and the benefits are profound.

"The physical benefits of Mediation are undisputed in the medical profession and include a reduction of stress levels, blood pressure and pain. Who wouldn't want those benefits? From a spiritual perspective, mediation is the primary method for enlightenment, anchoring energy and communication with higher consciousness and astral realms. Imagine tapping into the motherlode of information! Yes, you can!

"From personal experience and information from my Guides, I have learned that morning and evening 15 minute mediations are highly effective. In the morning, I set the intention to focus on instructions for the day. "Tell me what my tasks are today and how I may serve humanity." In the evening, I set the intentions I wish to see manifested. Remember to craft your intention as if it has already happened. "Thank you for helping me to solve my XYZ problem or thank you for healing my headache" It is critically important to word your request as a thank you for what is already done. Why? Because there is no time, no past, present or future. Time is a man-made construct. Einstein proved this.

Everything is happening in the now. Somewhere in the now your problem has been solved and you are thanking the Universal Presence for the solution. IT IS ALREADY DONE!

"Simple steps to begin a meditation practice.
1. Sit comfortably on the floor or in a chair. Place your hands at your side, in your lap or in lotus position.
2. Begin with breathing. Inhale deeply and hold for 7 seconds, Hold for 4 seconds. Exhale with an open mouth for 7 seconds
3. Imagine earth energy rising up through your body and exiting through the top of your head (Crown chakra)
4. Imagine the energy from the higher realms entering through the top of your head, moving down through your body and grounding into the earth.
5. Focus on the now. Push away all thought and mind chatter. This may take several attempts but keep trying. Some find it helpful to look into the flame of a candle to stay focused.
6. Get comfortable in the quiet of your mind. Allow images to come through but don't let mind chatter distract you. Don't fret if you don't get images. Listen for messages or just be still.
7. Feel yourself being connected to the Universe and all living things. Feel the joy, peace and harmony of this moment.
8. Feel yourself surrounded by violet light and feel it enter your brow Chakra, filling your 3rd eye.

9. Offer up your prayer for the day or intentions for the evening.
10. Slowly come back to your body and stretch before getting up.

"Remember that practice is the key. Keep focused and don't get discouraged. Add a few minutes to each attempt until you can stay centered for at least 15 minutes both morning and night. Keep adding time to your routine. Bravo if you can sit in meditation for an hour but don't be hard on yourself if you can't.".

APPENDIX V: GRATITUDE EXERCISES

This daily exercise is a must for me. In my opinion, gratitude is a must for a positive life and for a healthy mind, body and spirit. If you appreciate what you have, you do not want for much.

Studies have shown that practicing and feeling gratitude strengthens your relationships with your loved ones, increases your feeling of satisfaction with your life and encourages us to help others. Living in gratitude has been shown to increase happiness with one's life by at least 25%. Gratitude for me has driven me in my altruistic goals and my desire to help the planet and to help the people who help the planet and the animals of planet earth.

Living in the moment, in the now, is essential for a connected life. Most of us are raised to think of time as linear, with a past, a present and a future. However, in the spiritual universe, there is only now. All things are possible now and all things are available now. So the first part of a gratitude exercise is to root yourself in the now and try to ignore the past and the future.

Early in your day, try to think of what you are grateful for. You can do this before your meditation, in the shower or as you drink your morning tea. You can have as many or as few things as you wish on this list. Your list might consist of your spouse, your pets, your children, your friends, your job, the place you live, your parents or any number of things in your life. Your list can contain things and people, both large and small, in your life. You may be grateful for your cup of tea, your hot shower, the love that you have in your life. You might be grateful for the flowering Poinciana trees in June, for a spring rain, for the birds singing outside your window. The list is endless.

Now, every day, choose at least one or two of these and imagine for a few minutes, your life without these in it. Imagine that you have lost the love of your life to an accident or illness, and imagine your life without him or her in it. Now, imagine the pain that you feel at this loss. Allow yourself to feel the grief and pain. Now, bring that person back into your consciousness and allow yourself to feel the gratitude for this person and what they bring to your life, to your heart, to your being.

You can also imagine what your life might be like without your sense of sight, of sound, or the use of your legs. Try to imagine in detail your life without these senses and allow yourself to feel the loss and possibly, desperation at the loss of these abilities. Then bring the abilities back and fully feel gratitude for these wonders in your life.

Journal your gratitude. At the end of every day, or first thing in the morning, try to write five things from your day that you're grateful for. You can do this on your computer, in a notebook, or on your phone, for that matter. Focusing on these things will train your mind to positively embrace these things in your life and consciously appreciate the many joys in your life.

Be sure to tell those that you care for how much you love them. Never let an opportunity go by, because you never know when that may be your last opportunity in this lifetime.

Always thank those who help you, and do it consciously and with heart. When you say thank you, look into the person's eye and let them know that you truly appreciate their help. You will find that doing this will lift your heart and it will lift the day of those who you've thanked.

For the important people in your life, you may consider writing a gratitude letter from time to time, for 'no reason'. Let them know how important they are and what they've done that made a difference in your life. Be sure to thank them for being in your life and let them know how much you love and care for them.

As your day unfolds, try to take in everything in the day that you may have been ignoring. Go for a walk and really see the sky, the trees, the birds, and other wildlife. Smell the air, notice the smell of coffee or freshly cut grass. For everything that strikes your senses, give thanks and try to file it away in a special place in your heart and mind.

Try to help someone every day that you may have been ignoring. You may notice a homeless person that would appreciate a kind gesture. Offer help to an elderly person or someone who may seem lost or confused. Make eye contact and smile at strangers on the street. It's very easy to ignore those that might slow you down in your day, but sometimes taking the time to acknowledge these persons with simple gestures may be the difference between a good day or a bad one for them, and for you.

Once you begin to practice gratitude every single day, and begin to acknowledge the people, gifts, animals and things in your life that you are grateful for, you will find that you are happier in general, and when you are happier, you will begin to engage in healthier habits and thoughts.

APPENDIX VI: READING, VIEWING, PRODUCTS AND OTHER LIFE RESOURCES

This list includes books, movies and websites that have had a profound effect on my life and my wellness. As with all media, it's important to discern which of these or which parts of these are of benefit to you.

My notes are included with each, where applicable.

BOOKS:

"Healing and the Mind" - Bill Moyers (1993) This is available in hard back, paperback, audio book, Kindle edition and of course, there was a groundbreaking PBS series as well (available on DVD from PBS). While an older book, it is still valid today and it was more or less the first step for me in my understanding of the mind / body connection.

"Ageless", "I'm Too Young for This", "The Sexy Years: Discover the Hormone Connection: The Secret to Fabulous Sex, Great Health, and Vitality, for Women and Men" - Suzanne Somers

"The Hidden Story of Cancer" - Brian Peskin This book details the research of Nobel Prize winner Dr. Otto and refines it further, detailing the importance of a perfectly healthy cell. If cells are healthy, disease has no place to take hold. This is, by the way, a very large, very complex read. You will probably need to buy this book from Mr. Peskin's website.

"Grain Brain" - Dr. David Perlmutter   With the prevalence of Alzheimer's disease and other brain diseases in our aging population, this book presents a pathway to heal the brain and keep it healthy.

"Never Be Fat Again", Raymond Francis   This book was one of the 'jump starters' that fired my desire to stop the madness and heal myself.   Mr. Francis' own journey is inspirational and the simple fact that there are two things that will manifest wellness is the basis for his book: Add nutrition, remove toxins.

"Coconut Cures" - Bruce Fife, N.D. I found this on Raymond Francis' site **www.BeyondHealth.com** It is another handy guide that I consult for alternatives to drug store cures.

"Heal Your Body" - Louise L. Hay This is a convenient guide that I use when trying to determine if there is a mental or metaphysical component to a condition or illness.

"Archangels and Ascended Masters" Doreen Virtue   This is a wonderful reference.

"Love is in the Earth - A Kaleidoscope of Crystals" - Melody   This is another go-to reference for me.

"Thyroid Healthy" Suzy Cohen   Because of the

fluoride in our water, our food and in toothpastes, I believe that most Americans suffer from thyroid disorders, whether they test as such or not. This book offers a path to help your thyroid.

"Sex, Lies and Menopause: The Shocking Truth about Synthetic Hormones and the Benefits of Natural Alternatives" - T. S. Wiley

Dr. Otto Warburg, Nobel Prize winner for his work in cell health

MOVIES:

"Doctored" This documentary exposes the AMA, Western Medical community, Big Pharma and the FDA in an alarming way. My only concern is that parts of this movie appear to be an infomercial for the chiropractic industry. I have no real opinion of chiropractic myself but feel that it is an option that should be available to those who wish to take advantage of it. I personally chose to discard the pro-chiropractic portions and stick with the facts presented about the questionable activities of the FDA and the AMA.

"Food Inc" An alarming look at the food that we are sold in the US.

"Supersize Me" This film exposed the fast food industry as never before.

"King Corn" This film will spur you to eliminate

US grown, government subsidized corn and corn products from your diet. Since US corn and other grains such as soybeans and wheat is not accepted for import in Europe, Asia or even in Mexico, it begs the question as to why the people in the United States have yet to rebel against these toxic products.

PRODUCTS:

For aroma sprays: The Crystal Garden, Boynton Beach, FL. **www.TheCrystalGarden.com** I've used their sprays for years and have confidence that they're blended with love and guidance.

For aroma sprays and salts: Angel In Hawaii **www.AngelInHawaii.com** I have found her Archangel Ariel and Lakshmi sprays and salts to be very nice.

ABOUT THE AUTHOR

Suki S. Miller is a South Florida native and resident. She shares her life with her husband Mark, Siamese cats Mei Li and Mhysa and Yellow Nape Amazon parrot, Sophie.

CONTACT:

Email: **info@SukiSMiller.com**

Website: **www.SukiSMiller.com**

Please join our mailing list! Email the address above with your name, and email info. I promise we won't fill your inbox and we do not sell mailing lists.

Please visit our website for updates, promotions, specials and new books. Add your experiences and ideas to our blog.

'Follow' us on Facebook and recommend to your friends:

https://www.facebook.com/pages/Suki-S-Miller/403193023207981

Follow us on Twitter:
@SukiSMiller

Visit us on Goodreads.com:
https://www.goodreads.com/book/show/25973192-meditate-the-pounds-away

Manufactured by Amazon.ca
Bolton, ON